MEDITERRANEAN SIRTFOOD

|2 Books in 1|

The Sirtfood Diet + Mediterranean Diet Cookbook

The New Guide to Activate Your Skinny Gene, Burn Fat Fast and discover many tasty recipes of the original Italian Mediterranean diet | Over 120+ Quick & Easy Recipes + 28-Day Kickstart Plan for Lasting Weight Loss

|BOOK 1|

The Sirtfood Diet:

A Guide to Activate your Skinny Gene, Burn Fat, Lose Weight, and Stay Healthy with 50+ Easy Mediterranean, Pescatarian and Vegetarian Recipes! + 21days Meal Plan

|2021Edition|

Table Of Contents

Book 1: The Sirtfood Diet

Book 2: Mediterranean Diet Cookbook

MEDITERRANEAN DIET DINNER RECIPES 175

Mediterranean Diet Snacks Recipes 196

Conclusion 213

Introduction

This Diet relies on research sirtuins (SIRTs), a set of seven proteins utilized from the human anatomy that's been proven to modulate various purposes, including inflammation, metabolism, and life span.

Certain Natural plant chemicals could possibly find a way to grow the degree of those proteins inside the human anatomy, and foods containing them are known "sirtfoods."

The Diet blends sirtfoods and calorie limitation, both of which may possibly cause the human body to generate high degrees of sirtuins.

The Sirtfood Diet publication comprises meal plans and recipes to follow along; however, there are lots of additional Sirtfood Diet recipe collections out there.

The Diet's founders claim that after a Sirtfood Diet can cause accelerated body weight loss while maintaining muscles and protecting you in chronic illness.

Once You've finished the dietary plan, you're invited to keep on adding sirtfoods and also the diet signature green juice to your normal diet.

Thus Much, there aren't any persuasive signs that the Sirtfood Diet features a more favorable impact on weight loss than every other calorie-restricted diet regime.

Along with Although a number of those foods have healthy properties, there have yet to be any long-term human studies to ascertain if eating a diet full of sirtfoods has some concrete health benefits.

Nonetheless, the Sirtfood Diet publication reports the outcomes of a pilot study conducted with both the writers and between 3 9 participants in their exercise center.

Nevertheless, the consequences of the study appear never to have already been released somewhere else.

To get 1 week, the participants followed the diet and worked out each day. At the close of the week, the participants lost an average of 5 pounds (3.2 kg) and claimed even gained muscle tissue.

Yet These outcomes are hardly surprising. Restricting your own calorie intake to 1000 calories and exercising at the exact same period will almost always trigger weight loss.

No matter This type of fast fat reduction is neither true nor long-term, which analysis failed to accompany participants following the initial week to determine whether they attained some of the weight, and this is an average of the situation.

When Your own body is energy-deprived, it melts away its catastrophe energy stores, or glycogen, along with burning off muscle and fat.

Each Molecule of glycogen necessitates 3--4 atoms of water to bestow. Whenever your body melts away glycogen, then it eliminates the water too. It's referred to as "water".

The very first week of extreme calorie limit, just about one-fifth of those fat loss arises from fat, whereas one other two-thirds stems out of water, glycogen, and muscle.

When your calories grow, the own body accomplishes its own glycogen stores, and also, the weight comes back again.

Regrettably, such a calorie restriction may also cause the human body to reduce its metabolism, which makes it need fewer calories every day for energy compared earlier.

Additionally, it Is very likely that diet might help you drop a couple of pounds at the start, although it is going to probably return once the diet has ended.

As Much as preventing illness, three weeks might be long enough to own some measurable long-term effects.

The flip side, adding sirtfoods to a routine diet within the long-term, might just be a fantastic idea. However, in this circumstance, you may too, bypass the diet and begin doing this today.

Chapter 1: What Is Sirt Diet

Sirtfood Diet was developed in the United Kingdom by two nutritionists who were working at a private gym. They marketed the diet as a "revolutionary new diet" and health strategy that works by switching on the "skinny gene" in the human body system.

The Sirtfood diet is the latest way to burn extreme body fat and lose weight dramatically without having to experience malnutrition or starve oneself.

Activating the skinny gene is achieved through exercising and fasting. There are some categories of foods that have chemicals known as polyphenols that when consumed, they put little stress on the body cells. Thus, producing genes that imitate the consequences of both fasting and exercise. Certain foods have high polyphenols present in them such as dark chocolate (cocoa), coffee, red wine, kale and so on. When these kinds of foods are taken, they tend to release Sirtuins reactions that influence aging, mood and metabolism. Any diet high in Sirtfoods triggers weight loss without necessarily having to expend muscles, while at the same time maintaining a healthy lifestyle and health.

This particular diet focuses on calorie restriction which is in phases. This calorie restriction is believed to increase the production of Sirtuins in the body.

Is Sirtfood Diet Good for You?

Every food on the diet plan is very healthy for you. You stand to get the right amount of nutrients, vitamins, minerals and which will likely become high when following this diet. This diet is very restrictive on some kinds of foods and calories and this may make it a bit difficult for some people to follow and get accustomed to.

Is It Effective?

The developers of the diet are so positive about the wonders this diet performs in weight loss, in burning fat, in activating the body's skinny gene and in the inhibition of health-related conditions. The only concern is there's little proof to back these.

Conversely, there is no convincing evidence to ascertain the diet's beneficial effects on weight loss than any other type of food or diet restricted by calories. Nonetheless, many of the foods in this diet are rich in nutrients, minerals, and vitamins but there are no human studies to determine whether eating a diet high in Sirtfoods has any reasonable health benefits.

Contrarily to this, the Sirtfood Diet states the results derived from a pilot study the authors conducted which involved 39 participants from their gym. The result of this study was not published in any other source.

For the first week, the participants were put on a strict daily diet and exercise. By the end of the first week, the participants have recorded an average of 7 pounds weight loss. Achieving this result is not surprising at all, the reason being that restricting your calorie consumption to 1,000 calories coupled with exercise will result in weight loss.

Nonetheless, this kind of weight loss is not genuine and long-lasting. There was no evidence to determine if there was any follow up to know whether the participants gained back the weight, which is most likely to be the case. The key to this kind of diet is continuity. You have to keep following this diet until you have achieved your desired weight goal and then keep maintaining it over and over again. In the absence of this, the moment you make a sudden swerve from this diet, you are very much likely to gain those weight back.

When the body experiences energy deprivation, it utilizes either glycogen or its stored emergency energy and this is in addition to muscle loss and fat burning.

In a nutshell, Sirtfood Diet is likely to help you lose weight virtually because it's low in calories. But be prepared to gain the weight back once the diet is over. This is because the diet is very short to have a long-term effect on your body.

Sirtfood Diet Essentials

- *The diet consists of twenty highly rated foods, which you can combine with your everyday meal.*

- **Buckwheat**: *This is available in the form of noodles and fruit seed. It's in every way different from wheat. So, when getting yours, it should be 100 percent buckwheat.*

- **Celery:** *Very nutritious especially the hearts and the leaves. Always blend hem together.*

- **Extra virgin olive oil**: *This is a very top ingredient in SIRTFOOD DIET. It has a peppery taste and it's highly sirtifying.*

- **Bird's eye chili**: *Also known as Thai chili. They are hotter than regular chilis and have more nutrients.*

- **Capers:** *Good for salad.*

- **Green tea or matcha:** *Very soothing when combined with a slice of lemon.*

- **Cocoa:** *Helps in the control of blood sugar, cholesterol and blood pressure.*

- **Kale:** *It's a very high SIRTUINS activator. Rich in quercetin and kaempferol.*
- **Parsley:** *Sprinkle it on your meals, juice or smoothie. It's far more than just a mere garnish.*
- **Lovage**
- **Red onion**
- **Strawberries**
- **Chicory**
- **Turmeric**
- **Soy**
- **Red wine**
- **Walnuts**
- **Soy**
- **Medjool dates**
- **Rocket**

Does Sirtfood Diet Have Any Side Effects?

First and foremost, the diet has no room for substitutions. Sirtfood Diet is very limiting and restrictive. It counts calories and focuses on a certain food category.

Even though the SIRTFOOD recommended meals may look yummy and tasty, the diet is likely to be deficient in major nutrients like iron, zinc and calcium. They are not the kind of meal you will most likely find on the "list of healthy food" says an anonymous nutritionist. Eating a little bar of chocolate and having a glass of red wine is no bad thing and won't affect the body in any way. However, it shouldn't be an everyday thing. Eating varieties of fruits and vegetables is better and not just the ones recommended on the list.

Also, the weight loss can only be maintained only if the calorie restriction is also maintained otherwise, the weight comes right back. It takes time to burn fat and lose weight, there's no doubt about this. It's evident that this kind of weight loss is most likely to be that of fluid and not fat. The moment people go back to their former lifestyle and eating habit, the weight will be back in a matter of time, except if this is long term diet.

In essence, if you are not the type that skips food regulary, especially during the day, you are very much likely to experience some difficulties such as dizziness, headaches, nausea, inability to concentrate

Chapter 2: Why Everyone Talking About It

Propelled initially in 2016, the Sirtfood diet stays a hotly debated issue and includes supporters receiving an eating routine rich in 'sirtfoods'. As per the eating regimen's organizers, these exceptional nourishments work by enacting explicit proteins in the body called sirtuins. Sirtuins are accepted to shield cells in the body from kicking the bucket when they are under pressure and are thought to manage irritation, digestion and the maturing procedure. It's the idea that sirtuins impact the body's capacity to consume fat and lift digestion, bringing about seven-pound weight reduction seven days while looking after muscle. In any case, a few specialists accept this is probably not going to be an exclusively fat misfortune, however, it will rather reflect changes in glycogen stores from skeletal muscle and the liver.

Security and Side Effects

Despite the fact that the main period of the Sirtfood Diet is low in calories and healthfully deficient, there are no genuine security worries for the normal, solid grown-up thinking about the eating regimen's brief span.

However, for somebody with diabetes, calorie limitation and drinking generally squeeze for the initial scarcely any days of the eating regimen may cause risky changes in glucose levels.

All things considered, even a solid individual may encounter some reactions — essentially hunger.

Eating just 1,000–1,500 calories for each day will leave pretty much anybody feeling hungry, particularly if quite a bit of what you're expending is juice, which is low in fiber, a supplement that helps keep you feeling full.

During stage one, you may encounter opposite reactions, for example, weakness, dazedness and crabbiness because of the calorie limitation.

For the in any case sound grown-up, genuine wellbeing outcomes are improbable if the eating regimen is followed for just three weeks.

Sirtfoods are generally plant-based and high in cell reinforcements that help stunt your body into consuming fat at a higher rate. It's called Sirt on the grounds that it incorporates eating nourishments that are high in sirtuin activators, characterized as seven proteins found in the body that control digestion, aggravation, and the life span of cells. Created by two British Nutritionists, Aidan Goggins and Glen Matten, the nourishments should actuate your body's "thin quality" to consume fat quicker. They wrote the "official" direct: The Official Sirtfood Diet.

Why it works

Sirt nourishments help signal the body that it should fire up your digestion and increment bulk while you consume fat. Otherwise called superfoods, the main 20 sirtfoods incorporate the rundown underneath. Note that everybody gets amped up for the wine and chocolate however your body is entirely eating more fiber, more cancer prevention agents, and supplement thick nourishments.

Sirtuins Activate Your Body's Wellness Genes

People groups have consistently been interested in the 'Wellspring of Youth' and how we can live more and more advantageous lives. All things considered, established researchers have an equivalent interest with a group of qualities called sirtuins. All of us houses sirtuins—frequently alluded to as our thin qualities—and they are really entrancing, holding the ability to decide things like our capacity to consume fat and remain thin, our vulnerability to ailment, and even to what extent, we can live.

So, what makes sirtuins so ground-breaking?

Sirtuins are unique in light of their capacity to change our phones to a sort of endurance mode— setting off an incredible reusing process that gets out cell waste and consumes fat. The advantages of this are quite marvelous: Fat melts away and we become fitter, less fatty, and more beneficial.

So how would we exploit sirtuins?

This brings up the issue: What would we be able to do to actuate sirtuins and receive these stunning rewards? It is notable that both fasting and exercise initiate sirtuins. In any case, oh, both interest a steadfast duty to either food limitation or requesting exercise systems. Reducing calories leaves us feeling exhausted, hungry, and strongly cantankerous, and in the more drawn out term can prompt muscle misfortune and stale digestion. With respect to work out, the sum should have been powerful for weight reduction requires a LOT of exertion.

Both can be difficult to achieve.

In 2013, the consequences of one of the loftiest dietary investigations at any point did were distributed. The reason for the investigation, called PREDIMED, was flawlessly basic: It examined the distinction between a Mediterranean-style diet enhanced with either extra-virgin olive oil or nuts and an increasingly regular present-day diet. Results demonstrated that following five years, coronary illness and diabetes were cut by an unbelievable 30 percent, alongside significant decreases in the danger of weight in the Mediterranean eating routine gathering.

This wasn't unexpected, however when the examination was researched in more noteworthy detail it was found there was no distinction in calorie, fat, or starch admission between the two gatherings. How would you clarify that?

Not every (sound) food are made equivalent.

Research currently shows that plants contain common mixes called polyphenols that have colossal advantages for our wellbeing. What's more, when scientists dissecting PREDIMED examined polyphenol utilization among the members, the outcomes were faltering. Over simply the five-year time frame, the individuals who expended the most elevated levels of polyphenols had 37 percent less passing contrasted with the individuals who ate the least.

Be that as it may, not all polyphenols are equivalent. Information out of Harvard University from more than 124,000 people demonstrated that solitary certain polyphenols were useful for weight control. Also, an investigation of right around 3,000 twins found that a higher admission of just certain polyphenols was connected with less muscle to fat ratio and a more advantageous dispersion of fat in the body. Polyphenols are without a doubt a shelter for remaining thin and solid, yet in the event that not all polyphenols are equivalent, at that point which are the best? Might it be able to be those that exploration has demonstrated have the capacity to turn on our sirtuin qualities? Exactly the same ones enacted by fasting and exercise?

The pharmaceutical business has rushed to abuse these sirtuin-actuating supplements, contributing several millions to change over them into panacea drugs. For instance, the well-known diabetes medicate metformin originates from a plant and actuates our sirtuin qualities. In any case, up to this point they have been to a great extent ignored by the universe of sustenance, to the weakness of our wellbeing and our waistlines.

What nourishments initiate sirtuins?

With our advantage provoked we put all the nourishments with the most elevated levels of sirtuin-enacting polyphenols together into a unique eating regimen. This incorporates extra-virgin olive oil and pecans, the particular considerations in PREDIMED, just as arugula, red onions, strawberries, red wine, dim chocolate, green tea, and espresso among numerous others. At the point when we pilot tried it, the outcomes were shocking. Members shed pounds, while either keeping up or in any event, expanding their bulk. The best part is that individuals revealed feeling incredible—overflowing with vitality, dozing better, and with eminent upgrades in their skin.

Thus, the Sirtfood Diet was conceived, a progressive better approach to initiate sirtuins by eating heavenly nourishments. An eating routine that doesn't include calorie excluding, removing carbs, or eating low fat. An eating routine of incorporation in which you receive the rewards from eating the nourishments your adoration. The Sirtfood Diet is rocking the boat of good dieting counsel and what it truly intends to look and feel extraordinary. And all from eating our preferred nourishments!

Chapter 3: The Sirt Diet Plan

The nutritionists had developed the Sirtfood Diet. They were so interested in Sirtfoods' ability; they developed a diet focused on optimizing the consumption of Sirtfood and limiting mild calories. They then checked this diet on exclusive London workout participants and were shocked by their results. In the first seven days, gym participants dropped a total of 7lbs, despite not growing their workout rates. The participants not only shed a large amount of weight but also added strength (usually the reverse occurs while dieting) and registered major changes in physical health and well-being.

How the Sirtfood diet actually work?

The food is split down into two stages. Phase 1: the 'hyper success phase' of 7 days, incorporating a Sirtfood-rich diet with mild calorie restriction, and Phase 2: the 'maintenance phase' of 14 days, where you maintain the weight loss without reducing calories.

Is there any diet plan that exists for the Sirtfood diet?

Yeah, the is a handy map that shows you what you should consume every day, and when. It contains all the recipes that you'll require for the first three weeks. There's a meat/fish alternative for any day and a vegetarian/vegan choice. Nearly all of the meals are gluten-free, and dairy-free choices are accessible every day, ensuring that this is a lifestyle that should operate for most people.

What happens after finishing the Sirtfood diet?

The Sirtfood Diet is not meant as a one-off 'diet' but rather as a way of life. You are encouraged to continue eating a diet rich in Sirtfoods once you've completed the first three weeks and continue drinking your daily green juice.

How to do the Sirtfood plan?

The eating schedule describes the twenty foods that turn on the so-called 'skinny genes' to increase metabolism and energy rates. This simply stipulates you can lose 7lbs in 7 days.

The diet strategy will change the way you eat well. This seems like a name that is not user friendly, but it's something that you are likely to learn for a lot. Since the 'Sirt' is slang for the sirtuin genes in Sirtfoods, a community of genes called the 'skinny genes' that function, literally, like magic.

Eating certain items, the plan's developers claim, flips certain genes on, and mimics the results of calorie restriction, fasting, and exercise. It triggers a cycle of regeneration in the body, filtering out the cellular waste and garbage that accumulates over time and induces ill health and strength loss.

How does the diet work?

Sirtfoods function by triggering the body's so-called "skinny gene" receptors, the same genes that are triggered while we are exercising or fast. This makes the body lose fat in a manner that mimics the limit on calories, even without the lack of nutrients or other deficiencies.

The group of people studying the diet, including improved muscle mass and signs of feeling complete and happy with food consumption, showed an overall loss of 7 pounds of weight in 7 days.

Sirtfoods function as master regulators of our metabolism as a whole, most importantly having effects on fat burning while at the same time rising muscle and enhancing cellular health. Some of the items falling within the Sirfood grouping are also often aligned with the world's healthiest diets-such as the traditional Mediterranean diet. The program has two stages, with the first being the most intensive aspect of '7ibs-in-7-days' with the second going further at the side of things in terms of maintenance. The special foods trigger sirtuins (SIRTs), a group of 7 proteins found in the body which regulate the cycle of metabolism, inflammation, and aging. These specific proteins are believed to defend cells from dying due to stress. Researchers also conclude that sirtuins improve the body's capacity to lose fat and raise metabolism. Some plant compounds can increase the body level of those proteins. Foods that contain these compounds are called "sirt foods."

The possible cost of Sirtfood diets:

You just have to prepare and have access to the correct ingredients to adopt your diet properly. You will need to invest in a proper juicer too, which will run you at least $100. You will need to invest in some of The Sirtfood Diet collections, in addition to the free recipes available on the website.

The seasonality of products makes having strawberries and kale a little difficult at some periods of the year. Continuing on while driving, at social gatherings, and feeding a family of small children is always difficult.

The diet itself leaves off multiple food classes and is restrictive. Dairy products are not included on the menu and contain an assortment of important nutrients, including some that most people miss. Furthermore, the polyphenol-rich food matcha also contains lead in the tea leaves, which, particularly when taken regularly, is potentially harmful to your safety. Like 85 percent dark chocolate, it also has a deep and bitter taste, which is also suggested.

The bottom line:

Surely, polyphenol-rich products should be used in a weight-reduction plan, but they are not the foundation for a whole diet. Of course, you don't need everyday wine and dark chocolate, plus so much matcha is potentially harmful.

Detail of phase one:

The first phase continues for seven days, with calorie control and plenty of green juice included. It's supposed to improve your weight reduction and promise to help you drop 7 pounds (3.2 kg) in seven days.

The intake of calories during the first three days of phase one is limited to 1,000 calories. You consume three green drinks, plus one meal, every day. You will select from recipes here every day, many of which include sirtfood as a big part of the meal.

Detail of Phase Two:

Phase two requires two weeks to finish. You will begin to lose weight slowly through this "maintenance" period.

This stage has no clear calorie cap. Instead, you eat three sirt-food meals and one green juice a day. The meals are again chosen from the recipes included in any guideline.

After diet effects:

These two phases may be repeated as often as you wish for further weight loss. Nonetheless, upon finishing those stages, you are motivated to start "sirtifying" your diet by consistently integrating sirt foods into your meals.

There are a number of Sirtfood Diet publications, full of sirtfood rich recipes. You may also use sirt foods as a snack in your diet, or in recipes that you already have. You are also urged to start consuming the green juice every day. Therefore, the Sirtfood Diet is more a shift of attitude than a one-time diet.

Sirtfood diet plan does exist:

First week:

- *Limit regular consumption to 1k Calories.*
- *Drink three green sirtfood juices a day.*
- *Eat a meal rich in sirtfoods per day.*

Second week:

- Increasing your average consumption to 1.5k calories
- Drink two green sirtfood juices in a day
- Eat double meals per day rich in Sirt foods.
- There is not any fixed strategy at all in the long run. It's more about changing your diet to incorporate as many sirt products as you can, which will help you feel safer and more energy productive.

Chapter 4: The Sciences Behind Sirt Diet

Surely the diet will seem to work for certain individuals. In any case, scientific confirmation of any diet's triumphs is an altogether different issue. Obviously, the perfect investigation to think about the viability of a diet on weight loss (or some other result, for example, maturing) would require an adequately enormous example – delegate of the populace we are keen on – and irregular distribution to a treatment or control gathering. Results would then be checked over enough timeframe with severe command over puzzling factors, for example, different practices that may decidedly or adversely influence the results of enthusiasm (smoking, for example, or work out).

This examination would be constrained by techniques, for example, self-revealing and memory, however, would go some approach to finding the viability of this diet. Research of this nature, be that as it may, doesn't exist and we ought to, therefore, be wary when deciphering essential science – all things considered, human cells in a tissue culture dish presumably respond differently to the phones in a living individual.

Further uncertainty is thrown over this diet when we think about a portion of the specific cases. Losses of seven pounds in a single week are ridiculous and are probably not going to reflect changes to the muscle to fat ratio. For the initial three days, dieters spend around 1000 kcal every day – around 40–half of what a great many people require. This will bring about a fast loss of glycogen (a put-away type of starch) from skeletal muscle and the liver.

Yet, for each gram of put away the glycogen we additionally store roughly 2.7 grams of water, and water is overwhelming. So, for all the lost glycogen, we likewise lose going with water – and henceforth weight. Furthermore, diets that are too prohibitive are difficult to follow and bring about increments in hunger invigorating hormones, for example, ghrelin. Weight (glycogen and water) will therefore come back to typical if the desire to eat wins out.

As a rule, the use of the scientific technique for the investigation of sustenance is difficult. It is often unrealistic to do fake treatment-controlled preliminaries with any level of natural legitimacy, and the wellbeing results that we are often keen on happen over numerous years, making research configuration testing. Besides, considers in huge populaces rely upon shockingly shortsighted and guileless information assortment strategies, for example, memory and self-announcing, which produce famously inconsistent information. Against this foundation commotion, nourishment look into has a difficult activity.

Is There A Quick Fix?

Sadly, not. Sensationalized features and often a hyperbolic portrayal of scientific information brings about the apparently unlimited debates about what – and how much – we ought to eat, further fueling our fixation on a "convenient solution" or marvel fix, which in itself is an endemic social issue.

For the reasons sketched out, the Sirtfood diet ought to be entrusted to the prevailing fashion heap – at any rate from a scientific point of view. In light of the proof we have, to recommend in any case is, best case scenario fake and even under the least favorable conditions deceiving and harming to the authentic points of general wellbeing procedure. The diet is probably not going to offer any profit to populaces confronting a scourge of diabetes, sneaking in the shadow of corpulence. As expressed plainly by others, uncommon diets don't work and dieting, all in all is certainly not a general wellbeing answer for social orders where the greater part of grown-ups are overweight.

By and by, the best technique is long haul conduct change joined with political and natural impact, focused on expanded physical movement and some type of cognizant command over what we eat. It is anything but a convenient solution, yet it will work.

A diet that underlines dull chocolate, red wine, kale, berries, and espresso? It either seems like the most ideal street to wellbeing and weight loss, or unrealistic.

However, pause, it shows signs of improvement: According to the makers of the Sirtfood Diet, these and other supposed "sirtfoods" are indicated to enact the components constrained by your body's characteristic "thin qualities" to assist you with consuming fat and get more fit.

Bragging a rundown flavorful nourishment, you presumably as of now love, and supported by reports that Adele utilized it to get in shape in the wake of having a child, the Sirtfood Diet sounds naturally engaging.

Be that as it may, not to destroy your chocolate-and-red-wine high here, yet the science doesn't really bolster the diet's greatest cases. Which isn't to say that eating sirtfoods is an ill-conceived notion . . . yet, similarly as with all diets that sound unrealistic, you should take a gander at this one with the genuine examination. This is what you have to think about what sirtfoods can and can't accomplish for you.

As a matter of first importance, what the hell is a sirtfood?

Manufactured by U.K. Sustenance experts Aidan Goggins and Glen Matten, the Sirtfood Diet highlights plant-based feeding stuff known as "sirtuin activators." Basically, you animate the SIRT1 quality encoded proteins that Goggins and Matten called "thin quality" when you look at the key arrangement fixtures.

SIRT1 and sirtuin proteins are accepted to assume a job in maturing and life span, which might be identified with the defensive impacts of calorie limitation.

The case behind the Sirtfood Diet is that sure nourishments can actuate these sirt-intervened pathways sans the limitation, and consequently "switch on your muscle to fat ratio's consuming forces, supercharge weight loss, and assist fight with offing infection."

Alongside red wine, dull chocolate, berries, espresso, and kale, sirtuin-advancing nourishments incorporate matcha green tea, additional virgin olive oil, pecans, parsley, red onions, soy, and turmeric (a.k.a. phenomenal flavors and go-to solid treats).

There's some science behind the cases of sirtfoods' advantages, yet it's exceptionally constrained and rather disputable.

The science on the sirt boondocks is still very new. There are contemplates investigating the SIRT1 quality's job in maturing and life span, in maturing related weight addition and maturing related illness, and in shielding the heart from aggravation brought about by a high-fat diet. In any case, the examination is restricted to work done in test tubes and on mice, which isn't adequate proof to state that sirtuin-boosting nourishments can have weight loss or against maturing capacities in an absolutely real human body.

Brooke Alpert, R.D., creator of The Sugar Detox, says there's an exploration to recommend that the weight-control advantages of sirtfoods may come to some degree from the polyphenol-cancer prevention agent resveratrol, often advertised as a component in red wine. "All things considered, it is difficult to devour enough red wine to get benefits," she says, noticing that she does much of the time recommend resveratrol enhancements to her customers.

Also, some nourishment specialists aren't psyched about the way the Sirtfood Diet plan works.

According to top dietitians who've evaluated the arrangement, the Sirtfood Diet is feeling the loss of some significant components for a sound, adjusted routine. Goggins and Matten's diet plan includes three stages: a couple of days at 1,000 calories for each day, made up of one sirtfood-overwhelming dinner and green squeezes; a couple of long periods of two sirtfood suppers and two squeezes per day, for an aggregate of 1,500 calories; and a fourteen-day support period of sirt-y suppers and juices.

Keri Gans, R.D., creator of The Small Change Diet, says that she's "not wild about anything that runs in stages." Usually, the shorter stages make a hardship organize, which just prompts gorging eventually. "When you're limiting, anybody will get in shape toward the beginning of a diet," she clarifies. "However, we can't continue that eating design long haul."

According to Lauren Blake, R.D., a dietitian at the Ohio State University Wexner Medical Center, when you're hydrating and squeezing a great deal without a huge amount of calorie consumption, weight loss is normal, "however it's an ordinarily liquid loss," she clarifies. So, while one may shed beats on the diet, it's probably going to be impermanent and might have nothing to do with sirtuins by any means.

The decision? Sirtfoods are incredible to have in your diet, however, they shouldn't be all you have.

There's positively no explanation you can't include some sirtfoods into your eating plan, says Alpert. "I think there are some truly fascinating things here, similar to the red wine, dull chocolate, matcha—I love these things," she says. "I love mentioning to individuals what to concentrate on rather than what to nix from their diet." If it tastes liberal and it's solid in little amounts, why not?

Gans says she's an enthusiast of a ton of the nourishments on the sirt list, including staples of the Mediterranean Diet—the highest quality level of scientifically-supported smart dieting—like olive oil, berries, and red wine. "I can get behind nourishments rich in polyphenols and cancer prevention agents," she says.

Blake concurs that there's bounty to adore about the nourishments remembered for the diet, particularly the stylish fixings like turmeric and matcha that vibe crisp and help make eating fun and intriguing. "I'm seeing a great deal of plant-based nourishments that truly sparkle, and are loaded up with phytonutrients," she says. "Those are calming, and bravo."

Be that as it may, all the nourishment specialists recommend balancing the diet with some lean protein and sound fats, for example, progressively nuts and seeds, avocado, and greasy fish like salmon. Stir up your plate of mixed greens game, as well, with more kinds of veggies, spinach, and romaine lettuce notwithstanding the kale and red onions. Main concern? A large portion of the sirtfoods are An OK to eat and solid for you, yet simply don't depend on the diet to enact any "thin quality" right now.

Chapter 5: Activation of Sirtuins

What makes the Sirtfood Diet so strong is their ability to turn to an ancient gene family that exists within each of us. The name for that gene family is sirtuin. Sirtuins are unique in that they orchestrate processes deep within our cells that affect things as important as our ability to burn fat, our vulnerability to disease — or not — and ultimately even our life span. The influence of sirtuins is so deep that they are now called "the chief metabolic regulators." Basically, what exactly someone who wants to lose a few pounds and live a long and happy life will want to be in control.

In recent years, sirtuins have, unsurprisingly, become the subject of intense scientific research. The first sirtuin was discovered in yeast back in 1984, and research really began in the course of the coming three decades when it was revealed that sirtuin activation increases life span, first in yeast, and then all the way up to mice.

Why the thrills?

Because the basic principles of cellular metabolism are almost identical from yeast to humans and everything in between. If you can manipulate something as tiny as budding yeast and see a benefit, then repeat it in higher organisms like mice, there is potential for the same benefits to be realized in humans.

That takes us to fast. Consistently, the lifelong limitation of food consumption has been shown to increase the life span of lower species and mammals. This remarkable finding is the basis for the practice of calories restriction for some people, where daily calorie consumption is decreased by 10 percent, as well as its popularized offshoot, intermittent fasting, which has become a common weight-loss diet, made famous by the likes of the 5:2 diet, or Fast Diet. Although we are still awaiting evidence of improved longevity for humans from these activities, there is evidence of benefits to what we could call "healthspan "— chronic diseases are declining, and fat is starting to melt away.

But let's be honest, no matter how significant the advantages, fasting week in, week out, is a grueling business that most of us don't want to sign up for. Even if we do, most of us are not willing to stick to this. Besides this, there are disadvantages to fasting, especially if we follow it for a long time. We listed in the introduction the side effects of hunger, irritability, fatigue, muscle loss, and slowing in metabolism. However, ongoing fasting schemes may also put us at risk of malnutrition, impacting our well-being due to a decreased intake of vital nutrients. Fasting schemes are often entirely inadequate for significant proportions of the population, such as infants, pregnant women, and most likely older adults. Although fasting has clearly proven benefits, it's not the magic bullet we'd like it to be. This makes us ask, is this really the way nature was supposed to make us slim and healthy? There's definitely a safer way out there.

Our breakthrough came when we discovered that the profound benefits of calorie restriction and fasting were mediated by triggering our ancient sirtuin genes 5. To better understand this, it might be beneficial to think of sirtuins as the guardians at the crossroads of energy status and longevity. Therefore, what they do is to respond to stress in the body.

When energy is in short supply, there is a rise in tension on our cells, just as we see in the caloric restriction. The sirtuins sensed this, and then turned on and transmitted a series of powerful signals that dramatically altered the behavior of cells. Sirtuins ramp up our metabolism, increase our muscle's efficiency, turn on fat burning, minimize inflammation, and repair any cell damage. Sirtuins, in turn, makes us fitter, leaner, and safer.

A Passion for Exercise?

It's not just caloric restriction and fasting that stimulates sirtuins; exercise also does. Sirtuins orchestrate the profound benefits of exercise much as in fasting. But while we are encouraged to participate in routine, moderate exercise for its multitude of benefits is recommended, it is not the means by which we are expected to focus our efforts on weight-loss. Research indicates that the human body has developed ways of adapting naturally and that the amount of energy that we use while exercising, which means that in order for exercise to be a successful weight-loss strategy, we need to devote considerable time and effort.

That grueling workout regimen is the way nature intended us to maintain a healthy weight loss; this is even more questionable in the light of studies, now indicating that too much exercise can be harmful — weakening our immune systems, damaging the heart and leading to an early death.

Enter Sirtfoods

So far, we have discovered that triggering our sirtuin genes is vital if we want to lose weight and be healthy. Fasting and exercise have been the two known ways of doing this up till now. Unfortunately, the amounts needed for successful weight loss come with their drawbacks, and for most of us, it's merely incompatible with how we live twenty-first-century lives. Luckily, there is a newly discovered, ground-breaking way to activate our sirtuin genes in the best way possible: sirtfood. As we'll soon know, these are the wonder foods that are particularly rich in specific natural plant chemicals that have the power to talk to our sirtuin genes and turn them on. In turn, they mimic the results of fasting and exercise and, in doing so, offer impressive benefits of burning fat, muscle building, and health-boosting that were once unachievable.

Dealing with the Fat

One of the dramatic results from our Sirtfood Diet pilot study was not just the amount of weight the participants lost, which was very impressive — it was the sort of weight loss that really excited us. What caught our attention was the fact that a lot of people lost weight without losing any muscle. It wasn't uncommon actually to see people growing muscle. That left us with an inevitable conclusion: fat merely melted away.

Achieving a significant fat loss normally requires a considerable sacrifice, either severely reducing calories or engaging in superhuman exercise levels or both. Contrary to that, our participants either maintained or lowered their level of exercise and did not even report feeling particularly hungry. In reality, some even struggled to eat all of the food they had been provided with.

How is it even possible? Only when we understand what happens to our fat cells when there is an increased sirtuin activity, then we begin to make sense of these incredible findings.

Lean Genes

Mice genetically engineered with high levels of SIRT1, the sirtuin gene that causes fat loss, are leaner and more metabolically active, 1 whereas mice without SIRT1 are fatter and have more metabolic disease. 2 When we look at humans, levels of SIRT1 have been found to be significantly lower in obese people's body fat than their healthy weight counts. This is because we get benefits on several levels by sirtuins, beginning at the very root of everything: the genes that regulate weight gain.

To understand this further, we need to look deeper into what is happening in our bodies, which is causing us to gain some weight.

Fat Busting

We will explain this in terms of a drug-ring in Hollywood. The streets flooding with drugs is our body flooding with fat. The drug pushers on the street corners are the source of the weight gain peddling reactions in our bodies. But in fact, it's just the low-level thugs. The true villain is behind it all, masterminding the entire operation, directing every deal that the peddlers make. This antagonist is referred to in our film as PPAR-π (peroxisome proliferator-activated receptor-ÿ). PPAR-ÿ orchestrates the cycle of fat accumulation by switching on the genes needed to start synthesizing and storing fat.6 To avoid fat proliferation, you need to cut supply. Stop PPAR-ÿ, and you avoid fat benefit effectively.

Enter our hero SIRT1, who rises to bring the villain down. With the villain locked up tightly, there is no one to pull the trigger and the whole fat-gain enterprise crumbles. With PPAR-π's operation halted, SIRT1 is turning its focus to "cleaning the streets." Not only is this achieved by shutting down fat production and storage, as we have shown, but it is also altering our metabolism so that we begin to clear the body of excess fat. Like any good crime-fighting hero, SIRT1 has a sidekick, a central regulator known as PGC-1α in our cells. This effectively stimulates the formation of what is known as mitochondria. These are the tiny factories of energy that exist within each of our cells — the power of the body. The more we have the mitochondria, the more we can generate the electricity. But as well as encouraging more mitochondria, PGC-1α also encourages them to burn fat as the fuel of choice to make the energy. Thus, fat accumulation is blocked on the one side, and fat burning on the other increases.

Wat or Bat

We have looked so far at the effects of SIRT1 on fat loss on a well-known fat form called white adipose tissue (WAT). This is the sort of fat that weight gain coincides with. It specializes in storage and expansion, is stubborn, and secretes a host of inflammatory chemicals that prevent fat burning and further fat accumulation, rendering us overweight and obese. That's why weight gain always starts slowly but can snowball so quickly.

But the sirtuin story has another intriguing angle, involving a lesser-known type of fat, brown adipose tissue (BAT), which behaves quite differently. BAT is advantageous to us in full contrast to white adipose tissue and needs to be used up. Brown adipose tissue helps us expend energy and has developed into mammals to allow them to dissipate large quantities of heat-shaped fat. This is known as a thermogenic influence and is vital to help small mammals survive in cold temperatures. Babies also contain substantial amounts of brown adipose tissue in humans, but it declines shortly after birth, leaving smaller amounts in adults.

This is where the activation of SIRT1 is doing something truly incredible. It changes genes in our white adipose tissue to transform and assume the properties of brown adipose tissue in what is called a "browning effect."[8] This means that our fat stores begin to act in a radically different way — instead of storing energy, they start mobilizing it to be disposed of.

Sirtuin activation, as we can see, has an effective direct action on fat cells, allowing the fat to melt away. But there, it's not over. The sirtuins also have a beneficial effect on the most important weight reduction hormones. Sirtuin activation increases insulin activity [9]. This helps to minimize insulin resistance — the failure of our cells to react to insulin adequately — which is heavily involved in weight gain. SIRT1 also enhances our thyroid hormones' release and activity,[10], which share several overlapping roles in boosting our metabolism and, ultimately, the rate at which we burn fat.

Chapter 6: Calorie Restriction and Lifespan

Fasting-based diets have become very popular over the past few years. In fact, studies show that by fasting - that is, with moderate daily calorie restriction or by practicing a more radical, but less frequent intermittent fast - you can expect to lose about six pounds in six months and substantially reduce the risk of contracting certain diseases.

When we fast, the reduction of energy reserves activates the so-called "lean gene", which causes several positive changes. The accumulation of fat stops and the body blocks normal growth processes and enters "survival" mode. Fats are burned faster and the genes that repair and rejuvenate cells are activated. As a result, we lose weight and increase our resistance to disease.

The mysteries of thinness

Many studies have looked at the genetic specificities of overweight or obese people, Sadaf Farooqi, professor at the University of Cambridge, has chosen to focus on those of thin people. For this research, Sadaf Farroqi and his team worked with 1,622 thin volunteers, and used data from 1,985 severely obese people and 10,433 people of normal weight. Their DNA was collected and they answered a questionnaire on their state of health and their lifestyle.

Slimming is linked to genetics

The DNA study confirmed the results of other studies: certain genes have a role in the risk of obesity and have allowed new discoveries to be made, in particular, that other genes seem to be involved in slimming. The researchers gathered the data collected to develop a genetic risk index. "As we imagined, we found that obese people have a higher genetic risk index than people with normal weight," said one of the study authors. Conversely, thin people have a lower genetic risk index. 74% of the slim people in the study had slim and healthy people in their genealogy.

Target these genes to avoid obesity

"It's easy to make hasty judgments and criticize people for their weight, but science shows that things are much more complex, says Sadaf Farooqi. We have much less control over our weight than we would like". He now wants to push his research to identify precisely which gene influences thinness, this could help put the weight of specific treatment strategies for overweight people.

All this, however, has a price. Lower energy intake leads to hunger, irritability, exhaustion and loss of muscle mass. And the problem is precisely this with fasting-based diets: when they are followed correctly, they work, but they make us feel so bad that we cannot respect them. The question, then, is the following: is it possible to obtain the same results without having to impose that drastic drop in calories and, therefore, without suffering the negative consequences?

At this point, we just have to present you the Sirt foods, a group of newly discovered foods. These genes are sirtuins. They became famous thanks to an important study conducted in 2003, during which scientists analyzed a particular substance, resveratrol, present in the peel of black grapes, red wine and yeast, which would produce the same effects of calorie restriction without need to decrease energy intake. The researchers then found that other substances in red wine had a similar effect, which would explain the benefits of consuming this drink and why those who consume it get less fat.

This naturally stimulated the search for other foods containing a high concentration of these nutrients, capable of producing such a beneficial effect on the body, and studies gradually discovered several. If some are almost unknown, such as lovage, a herb that is by now very little used in cooking, the great majority is represented by well-known and widely used food.

The super regulators of metabolism

After the discovery of 2003, enthusiasm for the benefits of Sirt food skyrocketed. Studies reveal that these foods don't just mimic the effects of calorie restriction.

They also act as super regulators of the entire metabolism and burn fat, increase muscle mass and improve the health of the cells. The world of medical research was close to the most important nutritional discovery of the century.

Unfortunately, a mistake was made: the pharmaceutical industry invested hundreds of millions of pounds in an attempt to turn Sirt foods into a sort of miracle pill, and the diet took a back seat. We do not share a similar pharmaceutical approach, which seeks (so far without result) to concentrate the benefits of these complex nutrients of plant origin into a single drug. Instead of waiting for the pharmaceutical industry to transform the nutrients of the foods we eat into a miraculous product (which may not work anyway), we find it more sensible to eat these substances in their natural form, that of foods, to take full advantage of them. This is the basis of our pilot experiment, with which we intended to create a diet containing the richest sources of Sirt foods and observe their effects.

A point in common among the healthiest diets in the world

During our studies, we have discovered that the best Sirt foods are regularly consumed by the peoples who boast the lowest incidence of disease and obesity in the world.

Among the Kuna Indians, in the American continent, who seem immune from hypertension and with very low levels of obesity, diabetes, cancer and early death thanks to the intake of cocoa, excellent Sirt food, as well as in Okinawa, Japan, where a Sirt food, dry physique and longevity go hand in hand. In India, the passion for spicy foods, especially turmeric, gives good results in the fight against cancer. And in the traditional Mediterranean diet, which the rest of the western world envies, obesity is contained, and chronic diseases are the exception, not the norm. Extra virgin olive oil, wild green leafy vegetables, dried fruit, berries, red wine, dates and aromatic herbs are all effective Sirt foods, and they are all present in the Mediterranean diet.

Although Sirt foods are not a mainstay of nutrition in England today, the situation was quite different in the past. They were a basic element, and if many have become rare and others have even disappeared, we will soon see that it is possible to reverse the course.
For the first time, researchers have just highlighted a genetic cause of pathological thinness, associated with a risk of high mortality.

These studies, which point to the role of excess genes in underweight people who have difficulty eating, are published on Wednesday by the British scientific journal Nature.

The study, which involved 100,000 people, was led by Philippe Froguel (Imperial College / London and Institute Pasteur de Lille / France) and the Swiss team of Jacques Beckmann (University of Lausanne).

A fragment of chromosome 16 is known to be sometimes subject to fluctuations in the number of copies of its genes. The vast majority of people have two copies of each gene in this part of the chromosome, one transmitted by the mother, the other by the father. But about one in 2,500 people has only one copy (an under-dosage) and one in 2,000 has three copies (overdose of genes).

The Franco-Anglo-Swiss team had discovered in 2010 that the presence of a hole (a single copy) in this fragment of chromosome 16 could explain 1% of severe obesity.

It now demonstrates that people with an excess of genetic material (a "duplication") and therefore having three copies of this part of chromosome 16 have significant, even extreme thinness. They are up to 20 times more likely to be underweight than the general population.

These excess genes, 28 in number, are probably "appetite genes", underlines Professor Froguel. Thus, in children, half of the carriers of this anomaly are underweight and find it very difficult to eat. They can suffer from a developmental disorder and weigh at 4 years the weight of a child of a year and a half, said AFP Professor Froguel.

The researchers identified 138 carriers of the anomaly out of the 100,000 people studied. "In a third of the cases, this mutation was absent in the parents and in the remaining two thirds it was hereditary," notes Professor Froguel.

Example of female thinness: 1m60 for 40 kg (BMI of the order of 15). In adults of both sexes, "at 40 kg mortality is as high as in people who weigh 100 kg," he says. This genetic defect affects longevity: "There is no old man" in identified carriers.

The excess or deficiency of certain genes on the same fragment of the chromosome leads to opposite pathological consequences, underweight or obesity. It remains to clarify the mechanisms involved.

Of the 100,000 people studied, the researchers identified 138 carriers of the anomaly. "In a third of the cases, this mutation was absent in the parents and in the remaining two thirds it was hereditary," notes Professor Froguel. The region of chromosome 16 concerned by this duplication phenomenon comprising 28 genes, another step will be to identify which one has an impact on appetite and weight. It could be a single gene or a combination of several of them. This work also demonstrates that if certain genes from the same genetic region are present in excess (three copies) or deficiently (only one copy), this can lead, by a "mirror effect", to reverse pathological consequences - here the underweight or obesity.

Chapter 7: Foods to Activate Sirtuins

We've learned so far that sirtuins are an ancient gene family with the ability to help us lose weight, create muscle, and keep us super healthy. It is well known that through dietary limitation, fasting, and exercise, sirtuins can be turned on, but there is another innovative way to do this: diet. We refer to the most potent foods to activate sirtuins as Sirtfoods.

Beyond antioxidants.

To better appreciate the benefits of Sirtfoods, we need to learn about foods like fruits and vegetables very differently, and why they are perfect for us. Despite tons of evidence demonstrating that diets high in fruits, vegetables, and processed products usually cut the risk of multiple infectious illnesses, including the greatest killers, heart failure, and cancer, there is no denying that they do. It has been put down to their rich nutritional content, such as vitamins, minerals, and antioxidants, which is perhaps the best wellness buzzword of the past decade.

Yet this is a very different story we are here to share.

The explanation Sirtfoods is so amazing for you has nothing to do with the nutrients that we all know so well and hear about so much. Yes, they're all important items you need to get out of your diet, but with Sirtfoods, there's something completely different, and very rare. What if we threw the entire way of thought on its head and said that the reason Sirtfoods is good for you is not that they nourish the body with vital nutrients, or have antioxidants to mop up the damaging effects of free radicals, but quite the opposite: because they are full of weak toxins? This could sound insane in a world where almost every alleged "superfood" is actively promoted based on its antioxidant content. But it's a groundbreaking concept, and one worth taking on.

Sirtfoods may be a new culinary innovation, but it's obvious that throughout history, diverse societies have enjoyed their benefits. As we are more acquainted with the top twenty Sirtfoods below, we can see how many have been valued for their medicinal properties since early history, and have also been considered sacred foods for their ability to impart vigor and well-being.

Yes, it now seems that published evidence of these Sirtfoods benefits goes back a long way to being the subject of the very first clinical trial ever conducted. He was documented in Daniel in the Bible more than 2,200 years ago, we and him. It was considered the best food possible of the day and was recommended to keep the young people alive and eventually join the monarch's service. And, when Daniel opposed this, a plant-only diet yielded a better outcome in only a couple of days.

Such benefits should usually never be expected from a diet of only plants, particularly increased muscle mass. This, of course, is because certain plants were incredibly rich sources of Sirtfood. With reports revealing that the typical plants eaten back then were identical to the Sirtfood-rich conventional Mediterranean diet, and findings remarkably close to our pilot experiment, one can't help wonder whether the Daniel study is the stuff of fable, or do we unwittingly have the solution to achieving the body and well-being we've all desired for over two millennia?

Chapter 8: Top 20 SIRT Foods

The sirtfood diet comprises of a variety of different foods. The most significant benefit of a sirtfood diet is the wide variety of different food spectrum which can be incorporated in our personalized diet plan. The sirtfood diet can also have coffee and wine, which is the most popular reason that many celebrities are following this diet plan. sirtfoods are the most common and most widely used foods in both the Western and Eastern worlds. To be very specific, sirtfoods are those which contain high levels of a chemical compound called polyphenol. This compound is not uniformly distributed in sirtfoods, but every sirtfood contains specific amounts of polyphenols. You must be thinking that why only polyphenols are being tackled here. The answer is straightforward yet very informative. Polyphenols are the compounds that are present naturally in sirtfood, and many types of research conducted on these foods have confirmed that these foods have the highest impacts when losing extra pounds of fats from the body. However, the most famous foods in the sirtfood diet are actually twenty in number, and a significant portion of a sirtfood diet comprises of these superfoods. The reason to stick this food on a more significant proportion of the sirtfood diet is the higher number of polyphenols present in these foods, which is essential to unlocking the sirtuin gene in the body. This gene is arguably the most critical gene to trigger many fat loss cycles in the human body.

The top twenty sirtfoods are:

1. Arugula
The critical factor is the nutritious benefits provided by this food, which is rich in very unique and rare benefits. It is an outstanding food that can be used in health promotion and anti-aging. It is also called a superfood. A vast scientific literature is dedicated to supporting this food. It contains high amounts of antioxidants, antifungal, antiviral, disinfectant, and protecting benefits. It is also essential in the reduction of cholesterol from the body and thus reduces the chances of atherosclerosis and heart attacks.

A word Ramayana is used in traditional Indian medicine, which is associated with the global benefits of arugula in the human body. Arugula is a natural coolant that can be a protective remedy during hot summers. It also has cooling effects on the liver and stomach.

2. Buckwheat:

Stomach acids, disturbed gut mobility and injured food canal (esophagus) cause heartburn, a condition that affects every human many times in their lives. Buckwheat prevents heartburn by improving the capacities of the stomach and colon as well as by healing the food canal. Our large and small intestines have bacteria called E. coli, which are friendly in nature and help in digesting the food. Buckwheat is helpful to E. coli and thus improves the medium inside the large and small intestine. That helps to prevent irritable bowel syndrome and Crohn's disease, conditions that affect the colon adversely. It can effectively treat the issues related to constipation due to high concentrations of fiber.

3. Capers

The importance of this root plant in traditional Chinese herbalism is well known. It is considered a great root to promote the self-healing capacity of the body and to maintain vital forces inside the body. Some western herbalists also used this root as the primary source of tonic, which is essential to promote natural immunity and vital capacities of the body. This root has some fantastic impacts on neural and endocrinal systems of the body. It can be a primary herbal remedy for patients with deficient immunity or those who are treated by chemotherapy and radiotherapy.

These benefits of the herb make it an herbal remedy of choice for cancer patients all over the world. It is a primary adaptive herbal remedy in oncology. Moreover, the use of astragalus is hazard-free and safe. It has a fantastic impact on bone marrow, and thus, it can easily promote immunity by producing more potent white blood cells that can be used in the war against the deadly pathogens like bacteria and viruses. It is very high in concentrations of polyphenols, which help in reducing body fats from the body.

4. Celery

Much like to buckwheat, celery is very important for our stomach and intestine. Stomach acids, disturbed gut mobility, and injured food canal (esophagus) cause heartburn, a condition that affects every human many times in their lives. Celery prevents heartburn by improving the capacities of the stomach and colon as well as by healing the food canal. Our large and small intestines have bacteria called E. coli, which are friendly in nature and help in digesting the food. Buckwheat is helpful to E. coli and thus improves the medium inside the large and small intestine. That helps to prevent irritable bowel syndrome and Crohn's disease, conditions that affect the colon adversely. It can effectively treat the issues related to constipation due to high concentrations of fiber.

5. Chilies

Chilis are used in both western and eastern foods and can be utilized to achieve higher metabolic rates because these are rich in capsicum.

Capsicum is a potent fat mobilizer that can be used to break adipose tissues into much simpler precursors called fatty acid. Its action is dual. When these free fatty acids reach in our blood, the action of capsicum in chilies is to increase the basal metabolic rate, which is highly essential to burn these extra fatty acids in the bloodstream and thus promoting a lean physique without extra fat.

6. Cocoa

Cocoa is very important for the brain. By improving overall health and through its antioxidant properties, cocoa can reduce the chances of dementia, Parkinsonism, and much other related pathology. Fatigue is another crucial aspect to be tackled here. Mental fatigue is related to the exhausting of the brain after prolonged functioning or reduced brain capacities, which can lead to general body pains and low self-esteem. By providing the nutritional supply to the brain, cocoa can help to prevent the mental as well as general fatigue.

7. Coffee

Coffee is the reason for the popularity of the sirtfood diet. This diet regime allows the intake of caffeine in the body so that it can help in breaking the adipose tissues into fatty acid. Coffee, especially caffeine anhydrous, is beneficial in the mobilization of fats. Moreover, coffee also helps in reducing the fatigue in the brain, and it helps in the promotion of mental alertness. It is the biggest cause that the sirtfood diet provides mental focus and alertness to its users, which is not provided in many other ordinary fat loss diet plans.

8. Extra virgin olive oil

Olive oil is the most used type of oil throughout the globe. Italian and French diets primarily include olive oils in the main course. Extra virgin olive oil is the lightest form of olive oil. It provides many polyunsaturated fatty acids, which are actually high-density lipids. These fatty acids are essential in the reduction of blood cholesterol levels as well as they are a vital energy source in the body. Olive oil is well-researched about its benefits on the brain and cardiac health, and honestly, this attempt is not sufficient to describe the benefits of olive oil.

9. Green tea

Green tea is one of the most used types of tea around the world because of its health benefits. Green tea is well-researched about its benefits on the brain and cardiac health, and honestly, this writing is not sufficient to describe the benefits of olive oil. Green tea has rich historical importance in Indian ayurvedic medicine as well as in traditional western medicine. It was widely used to promote attention, focus, long-term and short-term memory, and brainpower in both children and adults. It was also used as an effective tonic for the heart and vascular health. In some literature, it is also shown that it was also used in lung diseases.

10. Red wine

The first evidence of grapes was found in Egyptian culture, and they were cultivated at the bank of Neil River. The literature is not complete to build a consensus that grapes were used in Egyptian civilization, but it is clear that they were very fond of wine even they were the first one who introduced it. So, it can be possible that they did enjoy the taste of red grape wine. However, history shows that once the drink was introduced, it spread at a swift pace over different zones of the globe, much like we are observing it today. In 55 B.C. after the arrival of Roman in British waters, they found locals enjoying a traditional cider-like drink, which appealed to them too, and soon, it was being considered as one of their favorite beverages. So, this beverage, with small changes in the recipe, was introduced in the Roman Empire and then to Europe. It was the most popular drink of Germanic heritage, and they added it to the Normans. When Normans defeated the British Empire in the 9th century, they brought the word "wine" into the English dictionary.

In many other fat loss diets, wine is a prohibited drink, but the sirtfood diet is unique in this regard. The sirtfood diet allows the use of red grape wine, and even it is an essential part of the sirtfood diet because of many health benefits assured by red grape wine.

Other foods which mark the top twenty list of the sirtfood diet are:

1)   **Garlic**
2)   **Kale**
3)   **Medjool dates**
4)   **Parsley**
5)   **Red endive**
6)   **Red onion**
7)   **Soy**
8)   **Strawberries**
9)   **Turmeric**
10) **Walnuts**

Chapter 9: The Potential Health and Weight Loss Benefits

Ecological factors significantly influence the destiny of living beings and sustenance is one of the most persuasive variables. These days life span is a significant objective of medicinal science and has consistently been a fabrication for the individual since antiquated occasions. Specifically, endeavors are planned for accomplishing effective maturing, to be specific a long life without genuine ailments, with a decent degree of physical and mental autonomy and satisfactory social connections.

Gathering information unmistakably exhibits that it is conceivable to impact the indications of maturing. Without a doubt, wholesome mediations can advance wellbeing and life span. A tribute must be given to Ancel Keys, who was the first to give strong logical proof about the job of sustenance in the wellbeing/sickness balance at the populace level, explicitly in connection to cardiovascular illness, still the main source of death overall. It is commonly valued that the sort of diet can significantly impact the quality and amount of life and the Mediterranean eating regimen is paradigmatic of an advantageous dietary example

The developing cognizance of the useful impacts of a particular dietary example on wellbeing and life span in the second 50% of the only remaining century produced a ground-breaking push toward structuring eats fewer carbs that could diminish the danger of constant maladies, subsequently bringing about solid maturing. Subsequently, during the 1990s the Dietary Approaches to Stop Hypertension (DASH) diet was contrived so as to assess whether it was conceivable to treat hypertension not pharmacologically. To be sure, the DASH diet was very like the Mediterranean Diet, being wealthy in foods grown from the ground, entire grains, and strands, while poor in creature-soaked fats and cholesterol. The awesome news leaving the investigation was that not exclusively did the DASH diet lower circulatory strain; however, it additionally diminished the danger of cardiovascular infection, type 2 diabetes, a few sorts of malignant growth, and other maturing related maladies To additionally improve the medical advantages of plant nourishment rich, creature fat-terrible eating routines, especially in hypercholesterolemic people, the Portfolio Diet was planned This eating regimen, other than being to a great extent veggie-lover, with just limited quantities of soaked fats, prescribes likewise a high admission of utilitarian nourishments, including thick filaments, plant stanols, soy proteins, and almonds. Curiously, members on the Portfolio Diet displayed a decrease of coronary illness chance related to lower plasma cholesterol and incendiary files in contrast with members on a sound, for the most part, vegan diet.

Nonetheless, additionally, the measure of ingested nourishment has been pulling in light of a legitimate concern for mainstream researchers as a potential modifier of the harmony among wellbeing and infection in a wide range of living species.

Specifically, calorie limitation (CR) has been exhibited to be a rising healthful intercession that animates the counter maturing instruments in the body.

In this way, the eating routine of the individuals living on the Japanese island of Okinawa has been widely broken down on the grounds that these islanders are notable for their life span and expanded wellbeing range, bringing about the best recurrence of centenarians on the planet.

Interestingly, the customary Okinawan diet came about to be fundamentally the same as the Mediterranean Diet and the DASH diet regarding nourishment types. Be that as it may, the vitality admission of Okinawans, at the hour of the underlying logical perceptions, was about 20% lower than the normal vitality admission of the Japanese, along these lines deciding an average state of CR.

In his most recent examination, showing up in the Aug8 print release of the diary Cell Metabolism, he saw what happens when the SIRT1 protein is absent from fat cells, which make up muscle versus fat.

At the point when putting on a high-fat eating regimen, mice coming up short on the protein began to create metabolic issues, for example, diabetes, much sooner than typical mice were given a high-fat eating routine.

"You've expelled one of the protections against metabolic decay, so on the off chance that you presently give them the trigger of a high-fat eating routine, they're considerably more delicate than the typical mouse."

The discovery raises the likelihood that medications that upgrade SIRT1 action may help ensure against weight connected illnesses. From that point forward, these proteins have been appeared to arrange an assortment of hormonal systems, administrative proteins, and different qualities, keeping cells alive and solid.

SIRT1 is a protein that expels acetyl bunches from different proteins, changing their movement. The potential focuses of this deacetylation are various, which is likely what gives SIRT1 its wide scope of defensive forces, Guarente says.

In the Cell Metabolism study, the specialists investigated the several qualities that were turned on in mice lacking SIRT1 yet encouraged a typical eating regimen and found that they were practically indistinguishable from those turned on in ordinary mice sustained a high-fat eating regimen.

This recommends in typical mice; improvement of the metabolic issue is a two-advance procedure. "The initial step is inactivation of SIRT1 by the high-fat eating routine, and the subsequent advance is all the terrible things that follow that," Guarente says. The scientists explored how this happens and found that in ordinary mice given a high-fat eating routine, the SIRT1 protein is cut by a compound called caspase-1, which is instigated by irritation. It's now realized that high-fat eating regimens can incite irritation, however, it's hazy precisely how that occurs, Guarente says. "What our examination says is that once you incite the fiery reaction, the outcome in the fat cells is that SIRT1 will be severed," he says.

That discovering "gives a pleasant sub-atomic system to see how fiery signals in fat tissue could prompt quick unhinging of metabolic tissue," says Anthony Suave, a partner teacher of pharmacology at Weill Cornell Medical College, who was not part of the exploration group.

Medications that focus on that incendiary procedure, just as medications that improve sirtuin action, may have some gainful remedial impact against heftiness related issues, Suave says.

Chapter 10: Empowering Yourself with Sirt Foods Building a Diet That Works

With the Sirtfood Diet, we've done something very special.

We've taken the foremost potent Sirtfoods on the earth and have woven them into a brand-new way of eating, the likes of which haven't been seen before. We've selected the "best of the best" from the healthiest diets ever known and from them created a world-beating diet.

The good news is, you don't need to suddenly adopt the normal diet of an Okinawan or be ready to cook like an Italian mamma. That's not only completely unrealistic but unnecessary on the Sirtfood Diet. Indeed, one thing which will strike you from the list of Sirtfoods is their familiarity. While you'll not currently be eating all the foods on the list, you presumably are consuming some.

So why are you not already losing weight?

The answer is found once we examine the various elements that the foremost cutting-edge nutritional science shows are needed for building a diet that works. It's about eating Sirtfoods within the right quantity, variety, and form. It's about complementing Sirtfood dishes with generous servings of protein than eating your meals at the simplest time of day. And it's about the liberty to eat the authentically tasty foods that you simply enjoy within the amounts you wish.

Hitting Your Quota

Right now, most of the people simply don't consume nearly enough Sirtfoods to elicit a potent fat-burning and health-boosting effect.

When researchers checked out the consumption of 5 key sirtuin-activating nutrients (quercetin, myricetin, kaempferol, luteolin, and apigenin) within the US diet, they found individual daily intakes to be a miserly 13 milligrams per day. In contrast, the typical Japanese intake was five times higher. Compare that with our Sirtfood Diet trial, where individuals were consuming many milligrams of sirtuin-activating nutrients a day.

What we are talking about maybe a total diet revolution where we increase our daily intake of sirtuin-activating nutrients by the maximum amount as fiftyfold. While this might sound daunting or impractical, it really isn't. By taking all our top Sirtfoods and putting them together during a way that's totally compatible together with your busy life, you can also easily and effectively reach the extent of intake needed to reap all the advantages.

The Power of Synergy

We believe it's better to consume a good range of those wonder nutrients within the sort of natural whole foods, where they coexist alongside the many other natural bioactive plant chemicals that act synergistically to spice up our health. We expect it's better to find out with nature, instead of against it. It's, for this reason, that point and time again supplements of isolated nutrients fail to point outlasting benefit, yet the exact same nutrient, when provided within the sort of whole food, does.

Curcumin is well established to be the key sirtuin-activating nutrient in turmeric, yet research shows that whole turmeric has better PPAR-γ activity for fighting fat loss and is simpler at inhibiting cancer and reducing blood glucose levels than curcumin in isolation. It's not difficult to ascertain why isolating one nutrient is nowhere near as effective as consuming it in its whole food form.

But what makes a dietary approach really special is once we begin to mix multiple Sirtfoods. For instance, by adding in quercetin-rich Sirtfoods, we enhance the bioavailability of resveratrol-containing foods even further. Not only this, but their actions complement one another. Both are fat busters, but there are nuances in how each of them achieves this. Resveratrol is extremely effective at helping to destroy existing fat cells, whereas quercetin excels in preventing new adipose cell formation. In combination they aim fat from each side, leading to a greater impact on fat loss than if we just ate large amounts of one food.

And this is often a pattern we see over and once again. Foods rich within the sirtuin activator apigenin improve the absorption of quercetin from food and enhance its activity. In turn, quercetin has been shown to synergize with the activity of epical catechin gallate (EGCG). And EGCG has been shown to find out synergistically with curcumin. Then it goes on. Not only are individual whole foods stronger than isolated nutrients, but by combining Sirtfoods we tap into an entire tapestry of health benefits that nature has weaved—so intricate, so refined, it's impossible to undertake to trump it.

Juicing and Food: Get the simplest of Both Worlds

Both juices and whole foods are integral to the Sirtfood Diet.

Here, we are talking about juices specifically made employing a juicer—blenders and smoothie makers (such because the NutriBullet) won't work. For many, this may seem counterintuitive, on the idea that when something is juiced the fiber is removed. Except for leafy greens, this is often exactly what we would like.

The fiber from food contains what are called non-extractable polyphenols (or NEPPs). These are polyphenols, including sirtuin activators that are attached to the fibrous a part of the food and are only released when weakened by our friendly gut bacteria. By removing the fiber, we don't get the NEPPs and lose out on their goodness. But importantly, the NEPP content varies dramatically counting on the sort of plant. The NEPP content of foods like fruit, cereals, and nuts is critical, and these should be eaten whole (in strawberries, NEPPs provide quite 50 percent of the polyphenols!). Except for leafy vegetables, the active ingredients within the Sirtfood juice, they're far lower despite an outsized bulk of fiber.

So, when it involves leafy greens, we get maximum bang for our buck by juicing them and removing the low-nutrient fiber, meaning we will use much greater volumes and achieve a super-concentrated hit of sirtuin-activating polyphenols. There is also another advantage of removing the fiber. Leafy greens contain a kind of fiber called insoluble fiber, which features a scrubbing action within the gastrointestinal system. But once we eat an excessive amount of it, a bit like if we over scrub something, it can irritate and damage our gut lining. Meaning leafy green–packed smoothies are going to be fiber overload for several people, potentially aggravating or may be causing IBS (irritable bowel syndrome) and hindering our absorption of nutrients.

Having a number of your Sirtfoods in juice form also can have big advantages when it involves absorbing their goodness. For instance, one among the ingredients we include within the green juice is matcha tea. Once we consume the sirtuin activator EGCG, found in high levels in tea, in drink form without food, its absorption is quite 65 percent higher. We also find it interesting to notice that once we ran blood tests on our own clients, switching from smoothies to green juices caused dramatic increases in their levels of other essential nutrients like magnesium and vitamin Bc.

The crux of it all is that to actually get those sirtuin genes to ring for dramatic weight loss and health, we'd like to create a diet that mixes both juices and whole foods for max benefit.

Go Big on Taste
A fundamental problem with conventional dieting is that it typically takes for a miserable dining experience. It drains all drop of delight from food, leaving us feeling dissatisfied.

But for us, it's essential that you simply maintain the enjoyment of food within the pursuit of a healthy weight. That's why we were delighted once we realized that Sirtfoods, also because the foods that enhance their activities like protein and omega-3 food sources, are primed to satisfy our desire for taste. It's the last word win-win: the Sirtfood Diet boosts our health and tastes great.

Let's take a step back to ascertain how this works. Our taste buds determine how tasty we discover our food, and the way satisfied we are from eating it. This is often done through seven major taste receptors.

Over countless generations, humans have evolved to hunt out the tastes that stimulate these receptors so as to realize maximum nourishment from our diet. The higher a food stimulates these taste receptors, the more satisfaction we get from a meal. And within the Sirtfood Diet, we have got the last word menu for happy taste buds because it offers maximum stimulation across all taste receptors. To summarize these tastes and therefore the foods you'll be eating on the diet that satisfies them: the seven major taste sensations are sweet (strawberries, dates); salty (celery, fish); sour (strawberries); bitter (cocoa, kale, endive, extra virgin vegetable oil, green tea); pungent (chilies, garlic, extra virgin olive oil); astringent (green tea, red wine); and umami (soy, fish, meat).

Crucially, what we've discovered is that the greater the sirtuin-activating properties of food, the more powerful y it stimulates those taste centers, and therefore the more gratification we get from the food we eat. Importantly, it also means we satisfy our appetite quicker, and our desire to eat more is reduced accordingly. This is often a key reason why those that follow a Sirtfood-rich diet are pleasantly fuller more quickly.

For example, natural cocoa features a striking, appealing bitter taste, but removes the sirtuin-activating flavanols with aggressive industrial food-processing techniques and that we are left with mass-produced, bland, and characterless cocoa that's want to make highly sugared chocolate confectionery. By now, the health benefits have vanished.

The same principle applies to vegetable oil. Consumed in its minimally processed form—extra virgin—it features a powerful and distinct flavor, with an invigorating kick that will be felt at the rear of the throat. Yet refined and processed vegetable oil loses all character, is mild and bland, and carries no such kick. Similarly, hot chilies boast much greater sirtuin-activating credentials than the milder varieties, and wild strawberries are much tastier than farmed ones thanks to a richer content of sirtuin-activating nutrients.

Not only this, but we also find that individual Sirtfoods can trigger multiple taste receptors: tea is both bitter and astringent, and strawberries have a mixture of sweet and sour flavors.

Initially, some palates won't be familiar with certain of those flavors—so much of our modern food is barren of both nutrients and true taste—but you'll be amazed how quickly you acquire a love for them. After all, humans evolved to hunt out a diet rich in Sirtfoods, alongside healthful protein and omega-3 fatty acids, to satisfy the essential desires of our appetite and, in turn, our health. This evolutionary process occurred over millennia, without us knowing the explanations, yet it ensured we got maximum to enjoy consuming these foods.

Chapter 11: How to Follow the Sirt Diet

Phase One and Phase Two?

The Sirtfood diet consists of two phases. I have to warn you, the first week of food is the hardest part. And you need to focus on the end of the first week, especially the early three days. Don't worry; the long-term plan is easy to follow and maintain.

The First Step

This level is divided into two levels (days 1, 2 and 3 / days 4, 5, 6 and 7).

For days 1, 2 and 3, dieters should consume two green juices per day (including green tea, parsley, lemon, celery, arugula and kale) and only one meal. You should limit your intake to just 1,000 calories a day.

I call this the detox/quick/juice phase, and it is generally intended for those who want to accelerate weight loss. The key, of course, is that every juice or meal contains Sirtfood ingredients.

To cope with the first three days, just keep an eye on the goal: lighter weight and a healthier body. And don't worry, the green juice is not that bad (I like these green juices). They also have a sumptuous dinner and can even make dark chocolates to appease your treats.

The second phase

Congratulations! You have completed the first week of "Hardcore".

The second phase is the simplest and consists of including sirtuin-based foods in your diet or your daily meals. You can call this the "maintenance phase".
In this way, your body goes through the stage of burning fat and building muscle, as well as strengthening your immune system and your general health.
In this phase, you can now eat three balanced meals with Sirtfood plus one green juice per day.

There is no "diet", but the choice of healthier alternatives by adding Sirtfood to each meal as often as possible.

Then, I will provide delicious cooking recipes with Sirtfood to give you an idea of the excitement and health of this diet trip.

What are sirtuins?

Sirtuins, or SIRT for short, belong to the family of proteins that regulate cell health, including homeostasis. Hemostasis is the process by which the body maintains its stability and adjusts the conditions most conducive to its survival.

The SIRT family of proteins includes seven members (SIRT1-7). The yeast mute information regulator SIR2 is the founding member of the SIRT family of proteins, which controls chromatin, DNA recombination and gene expression.

Among the seven mammalian SIRTs, SIRT1, SIRT2 and SIRT3 have a deacetylase capacity. The other remaining SIRTs (SIRT4, SIRT5, SIRT6 and SIRT7) have weak or undetectable deacetylate activity. SIRT1-7 differ in their function and location.

SIRT1 is located in the cytosol and in the cell nucleus, where it fulfils its cell life function. It is involved in glucose metabolism, neurodegeneration, differentiation, control of gene expression, ageing, cell death and tumor development. SIRT2 is in the cytosol and catalyzes the deacetylation of alpha-tubulin (Lys40), H31ys56, FOXO1, H41ys16 and FOXO3a. Also, it is involved in the regulation of gene expression, tubulin acetylation, tubulin acetylation, cell cycle regulation, response to DNA damage, cancer and neurodegeneration...

Localization of SIRT3 on the inner membrane of the mitochondria with long-chain substrates acyl-CoA dehydrogenase (LCDA), acetyl-CoA synthetase 2 (ACS2), 2,3-hydroxy-3-methyl glutaryl CoA synthetase 2 (HMGCS2), ornithine Transcarbamoyl transferase (OTC), glutamate dehydrogenase (GDH), cycle-Philip D, superoxide dismutase 2 (SOD2), Isocitrate dehydrogenase 2 (IDH2), many components of the respiratory chain complexes of mitochondria and Ku70. It is responsible for the production of mitochondrial ATP, the oxidation of fatty acids and the regulation of mitochondrial protein. It also controls caloric restriction and cellular response to oxidative stress by activating SOD2 and IDH2, which in turn reduces oxidized reactive oxygen species (ROS) and glutathione. It is also involved in the suppression of tumors and cell death, which has a positive impact on genomic stability. SIRT4 is in the mitochondrial matrix. It is engaged in the ribosylation of ADP and inhibition of GHD using NAD +.

SIRT5, it is also found in the mitochondrial matrix and contains a decarboxylase dependent on NAD + and the succinyls activity in CPS1.

SIRT6, which acts as a deacetylase and ADP ribosyltransferase, is necessary for telomeric functions, hemostasis of metabolism, DNA repair and genome stability.

SIRT7 is mainly a nucleolar protein which regulates the transcription of ribosomal genes by interaction with RNA polymerase 1. SIRT7 has a high selectivity for H3lys18 and a deacetylase dependent on NAD +. When SIRT7 is deacetylated, we must suppress the genes involved in cell anchoring and inhibit contact, thus promoting the malignant phenotype of tumor cells. As well as desuccinylase activity in CPS1. SIRT6, which acts as a deacetylase and ADP ribosyltransferase, is necessary for the functions of telomeres, hemostasis of metabolism, DNA repair and genome stability. SIRT7 is mainly a nucleolar protein which regulates the transcription of ribosomal genes by interaction with RNA polymerase 1.

SIRT7 has a high selectivity for H3lys18 and a deacetylase dependent on NAD +. When SIRT7 is deacetylated, we need to suppress the genes involved in cell anchoring and inhibit contact, thus promoting the malignant phenotype of tumor cells. As well as the desuccinylase activity in CPS1. SIRT6, which acts as a deacetylase and ADP ribosyltransferase, is necessary for telomeric functions, hemostasis of metabolism, DNA repair and genome stability. SIRT7 is mainly a nucleolar protein, which regulates the transcription of ribosomal genes by interaction with RNA polymerase 1. SIRT7 has a high selectivity for H3lys18 and a deacetylase dependent on NAD +. When SIRT7 is deacetylated, we must suppress the genes involved in cell anchoring and inhibit contact, thus promoting the malignant phenotype of tumor cells.

Genome stability. SIRT7 is mainly a nucleolar protein which regulates the transcription of ribosomal genes by interaction with RNA polymerase 1. SIRT7 has a high selectivity for H3lys18 and a deacetylase dependent on NAD +. When SIRT7 is deacetylated, we need to suppress the genes involved in cell anchoring and inhibit contact, thus promoting the malignant phenotype of tumor cells.

Genome stability. SIRT7 is mainly a nucleolar protein which regulates the transcription of ribosomal genes by interaction with RNA polymerase 1. SIRT7 has a high selectivity for H3lys18 and a deacetylase dependent on NAD +. When SIRT7 is deacetylated, we need to suppress the genes involved in cell anchoring and inhibit contact, thus promoting the malignant phenotype of tumor cells.

The science of sirt food

The sirt diet cannot be classified as low in carbohydrates or low in fat. This diet is very different from its many predecessors and at the same time advocates many of the same things: eating fresh plant foods. As the name suggests, it is a diet based on sirtuins. But what are sirtuins, and why have you never heard of them?

There are seven Sirtuin proteins: SIRT-1 to SIRT-7a. They can be found in all cells and the cells of all animals on the planet. Sirtuins are found in almost all living organisms and nearly all parts of the cell and control what happens. The supplement company Elysium Health compares body cells to an office with sirtuins, which act as CEOs and help cells respond to internal and external changes. They regulate what is done when it is done and who does it.

Of the seven sirtuins, one acts in the cytoplasm of your cell, three in the mitochondria of the cell and three in the cell nucleus. They are busy, but they mainly eliminate acetyl groups from other proteins. These acetyl groups indicate that the protein to which they are attached is available to perform its function. The sirtuins remove the available flag and prepare the protein for use. Sirtuins seem quite crucial for the normal functioning of your body. Why have you never heard of it?

The first sirtuin discovered was SIR2, a gene found in the 1970s which controlled fruit flies' ability to mate. It wasn't until the 1990s when scientists discovered other similar proteins in nearly all life forms. Each organism had a different amount of sirtuins: one has bacteria and five has yeast. Mice experiments show that they have seven, the same number as humans.

Sirtuins have proved to prolong the yeasts and mice's life. So far, there is no evidence of the same effect in humans, but in almost all forms of life these sirtuins are present, and many scientists hope that organisms as distant as yeast and mice will have the same effect as sirtuins. Activation may be extended to humans, too.

In addition to sirtuins, our body needs another substance called.
Nicotinamide adenine dinucleotide for cells to function correctly. Elysium (see above) compares this substance to the money a business needs to keep it going. Like any CEO, a sirtuin can only manage the business properly if there is sufficient cash flow. NAD + was first discovered in 1906. You get your diet from NAD + from your diet by eating foods made from the building blocks of NAD +.

Chapter 12: Succeeding with Phase One

This is the period of hyper-success, where you will take a massive move in creating a slimmer, leaner body. Follow our easy step-by-step directions and use the delicious recipes you'll find. We also have a meat-free version in addition to our regular seven-day schedule, which is suitable for vegetarians and vegans alike. Feel free to go along with whatever you want.

What to Expect

You'll enjoy the full benefits of our clinically proven strategy of dropping 7 pounds in seven days during Phase 1. Yet note that involves adding strength, so don't hang up simply with the percentages on the scales. Nor should you become used to measuring yourself every day. In reality, in the last few days of Phase 1, we often see the scales rising due to muscle growth, although waistlines continue to shrink. So, we want you to look at the charts, but not be controlled by them. Find out how you feel inside the mirror, if your clothes fit, or if you need to push a knot on your belt. These are all perfect measures of the underlying shifts in your body composition.

Be mindful of other improvements, too, such as wellbeing, energy levels, and how smooth the skin is. In a local pharmacy, you can even get tests of your general cardiovascular and metabolic wellbeing to see improvements in factors like your blood pressure, blood sugar levels, and blood fats like cholesterol and triglycerides. Also, weight loss aside, incorporating Sirtfoods into your diet is a big step in making your cells fitter and more disease prone, setting you up for an extraordinary balanced lifetime.

How to Follow Phase 1

We will lead you through the full seven-day program one day at a time to make Phase 1 as plain sailing as possible, including the lowdown on the Sirtfood green juice and easy-to-follow, delicious recipes every step of the way.

This phase of Sirtfood Diet has two different stages:

Days 1 to 3 are the most important and you can eat up to a limit of 1000 calories every day during this time, consisting of:

➢ Three times Sirtfood green juices
➢ One main course

Days 4 to 7 will see the daily intake of food rise to a maximum of 1,500 calories, composed of:

➢ Two times Sirtfood green juices

> ➢ Two main courses

There are very few laws with which to obey the diet. Mostly, for lasting progress, it's about incorporating it into the lifestyle and around everyday life. But here are a few easy but big impact tips to get the best result:

1. Take a Good Juicer
Juicing is an essential aspect of the Sirtfood Diet, and a juicer is one of the best health-care purchases you can make. Although price should be the determining factor, certain juicers are more effective at extracting the juice from green leafy vegetables and herbs, with the Breville brand among the best juicers we've tested.

2. Start Preparation
One thing is clear from the multitude of feedback we've had: those who planned ahead of time were the most successful. Get to know the products and techniques, and stock up on what's essential. You'll be amazed at how natural the whole cycle is, with everything planned and ready.

3. Save your Important Time
When time is tight, dress cleverly. Meals can be made the other night. Juices can be produced in bulk and stored in the refrigerator for up to three days (or longer in the freezer) until their sirtuin-activating nutrient levels begin to fall. Only shield it from light, and only add when you're able to eat it in the match.

4. Eat Early
Eating early in the day is healthier, and hopefully, meals and drinks should not be consumed after 7 p.m. But the plan is primarily designed to fit the lifestyle, and late eaters always enjoy great benefits.

5. Space Out the Juices
These should be taken at least one hour before or two hours after a meal to maximize the digestion of the green juices and dispersed throughout the day, rather than making them very close together.

6. Eat till You Feel Satisfied
Sirtfood can have dramatic effects on appetite, and some individuals will be satisfied before their meals are over. Hear your body and feed until you're full, instead of forcing down all the calories. Because Okinawans have existed for a long time, it states, "Feed before 80 percent full."

7. Enjoy the Diet

Don't get caught up on the end goal but keep aware of the road instead. This lifestyle is about enjoying food in all its glory, for its health benefits but also for the fun and pleasure it offers. Research shows that we are far more likely to succeed if we maintain our eyes focused on the road rather than the final destination.

Drinks

As well as the recommended daily portions of green beverages, other drinks can be easy drinking in Phase 1. Non-calorie beverages, usually regular juice, black coffee, and green tea. If your usual tastes are for black or herbal teas, do not hesitate to include these too. Fruit juices and soft drinks are left behind.

Alternatively, try adding a few sliced strawberries to still or sparkling water to make your Sirtfood-infused health drink, if you want to spice things up. Hold it for a few hours in the fridge, and you will have a surprisingly cooling option to soft drinks and juices.

One aspect that you have to be aware of is that we don't suggest abrupt, significant changes to your daily use of coffee. Symptoms of caffeine withdrawal can make you feel bad for a few days; similarly, significant increases can be painful for those particularly sensitive to caffeine results. They also recommend drinking coffee without adding milk, because some researchers have found that adding milk will decrease the absorption of the beneficial sirtuin-activating nutrients. The same has been observed with green tea but incorporating any lemon juice increases the absorption of its sirtuin-activating nutrients.

Note that this is the period of hyper-success, and while you should be comforted by the knowledge that it is only for a week, you need to be a little more careful. We have alcohol for this week, in the form of red wine but only as a cooking component.

The Sirtfoods Green Juices

The green juice is an essential part of the Sirtfood Diet's Phase 1 program. All the ingredients are strong Sirtfoods, and in every juice, you get a potent mixture of natural compounds like apigenin, kaempferol, luteolin, quercetin, and EGCG that function together to turn on your sirtuin genes and encourage fat loss. To that, we have attached lemon, as it has been shown that its natural acidity prevents, stabilizes, and improves the absorption of the sirtuin-activating nutrients. We added a touch of apple and ginger to taste too. But both of these are available. Nevertheless, several people find that they take the apple out entirely once they are used to the flavor of the fruit.

Sirtfood Green Juices (SERVES 1)

• Two handfuls (about two and a half ounces) kale
• A handful (one ounce or 30g) arugula
• A small handful (about one-fourth ounce or 5g) parsley leaves
• Two to three large celery stalks (five and a half ounces or 150g), including leaves
• Half medium green apple
• Half - to One-inch (1 to 2.5 cm) piece of fresh ginger
• Juice of a half lemon
• Half teaspoon matcha powder*
*Days 1 to 3 of Phase 1: added only to the first two juices of the day
*Days 4 to 7 of Phase 1: added to both juices

Remember that while we weighted all the amounts precisely as described in our pilot experiment, our experience is that a handful of measures work exceptionally well. In reality, they are the best tailoring the number of nutrients to the body size of a person. More significant people tend to have more massive paws, and thus get a proportionally higher volume of Sirtfood nutrients to suit their body size and vice versa for smaller people.

• Bring together the greens (kale, arugula, and parsley), and blend them. We consider juicers may vary in their efficacy when juicing leafy vegetables, and you may need to re-juice the remains before going on to the other ingredients. The goal is to end up with around 2 ounces of material, or about 1/4 cup (50ml) of green juice.
• Now, blend the Celery, apple, and ginger.
• You should cut the lemon and also bring it through the juicer, but we find it much easier to push the lemon into the juice by hand. You should have about 1 cup (250ml) of juice in total by this point, perhaps somewhat more.
• It's only when you extract the juice and are ready to serve that you add the matcha. In a bowl, pour a tiny amount of juice, then add the matcha, and mix vigorously with a fork or whisk. In the first two beverages of the day, we only use matcha, because it includes small amounts of caffeine (the same quality as a regular teacup). When wasted late, it can keep you awake with those not used to it.
• After the matcha is resolved, add the juice that left. Give it a final blend, and the juice is ready to drink. Easy to top up with plain water, as you like.

Chapter 13: Research Your Goal in Phase Two

Congratulations on completing Sirtfood Diet Step 1! You will already see amazing results with a weight loss and not only look slimmer and more toned but also feel revitalized and re-energized.

So, now what?

Having seen these often-remarkable transformations firsthand ourselves, we know how much you're going to want to see even better results, not just preserve all those benefits. Sirtfoods are, after all, designed to eat for life. The problem is how you adapt what you did in Phase 1 into your normal dietary routine. That's exactly what prompted us to develop a fourteen-day maintenance plan designed to help you make the transition from Phase 1 to your more usual dietary routine, thus helping to maintain and expand the Sirtfood Diet's benevolence.

What to Expect
You should maintain your weight-loss results during Phase 2, and continue to lose weight gradually.

Also, the one striking thing we've found with the Sirtfood Diet is that most or all of the weight people lose is from fat and that many actually put some muscle in.
So, we would like to remind you again not to measure your success solely on the scale by the numbers. Look in the mirror to see if you look leaner and more toned, see how your clothes are tingling, and lap up the compliments you're going to get from others.

Remember also that as the weight loss continues, so will the health benefits increase. By following the 14-day maintenance plan, you are really starting to lay the foundations for a lifelong health future.

How to Follow Phase 2
The key to success in this process is keeping your diet filled with Sirtfoods. To make it as simple as possible, we have prepared a seven-day menu plan for you to follow, including delicious family-friendly recipes, filled with Sirtfoods every day to the rafters (although see page 149 for children's advice). All you need to do is repeat the Seven Day Plan twice to complete Phase 2's fourteen days.

On each of the fourteen days, your diet will consist of:

• 3 x balanced sirtfood-rich meals

• 1 x sirtfood green juice
• 1 to 2 x optional snacks Sirtfood bite snacks

Once again, when you have to consume these, there are no rigid rules. Be flexible throughout your day, and t them. Two simple thumb rules are: • Have your green juice either in the morning, at least 30 minutes before breakfast, or in the middle of the morning. • Do your hardest to eat your dinner by 7 p.m.

Portion SIZES
During Phase 2, our attention is not on calorie counting. For the average person, this is not a practical approach or even a successful one over the long term.

Alternatively, we concentrate on small servings, really well-balanced meals, and, most importantly, filling up on Sirtfoods so that you can continue to enjoy their fat burning and health-promoting effects.

We've also designed the meals in the plan to make them satiate, making you feel satisfied for longer. That, combined with Sirtfoods' natural appetite-regulating effects, means you're not going to spend in 14 days feeling hungry, but rather happily satisfied, well-fed, and extremely well-fed.

Just like in Phase 1, remember to listen and be guided by your appetite. If you make meals according to our instructions, and you are comfortably full before you have a meal, then stop eating is perfectly fine!

What to Drink
In phase 2, you can need to have one green juice per day. This is to keep you top with high Sirtfoods levels.

Just as in Phase 1, during Phase 2, you can freely ingest other fluids. Our favorite beverages include remaining plain water, homemade flavored beer, coffee, and green tea. If black or white tea is your predilection, feel free to enjoy it. The same goes for herbal teas. The best news is that during Phase 2, you can enjoy the occasional glass of red wine. Because of its sirtuin-activating polyphenols content, especially resveratrol and piceatannol, red wine is a sirt food which makes it by far the best alcoholic beverage choice. But, with alcohol itself having adverse effects on our fat cells, moderation is still best and we recommend that you limit your intake for two or three days a week to one glass of red wine with a meal during Phase 2.

Chapter 14: How to Continue Managing Your Weight Returning to Three Meals

You ate only one or two meals a day during Phase 1, which gave you plenty of leisure time to eat your meals. As we are now returning to a more usual schedule and the time-tested practice of three meals a day, thinking about breakfast is a good time.

Eating a healthy breakfast will make us ready for the day and will increase our strength and focus. Eating earlier, in terms of metabolism, keeps our blood sugar and fat levels in check. Several studies have borne out that breakfast is a good thing, typically showing people who regularly eat breakfast are less likely to get overweight.

That is because of our internal body clocks. Our bodies are expecting us to eat early in anticipation of when we will be most busy and need food. Yet as many as a thirds of us will miss breakfasts on any given day. It's a classic symptom of our busy modern life, and the impression is there's simply not enough time to eat well. But as you will see, nothing could be further from the truth with the nifty breakfasts that we have laid out here for you. Whether it's the Sirtfood smoothie that can be drunk on the go, the premade Sirt muesli or the fast and easy Sirtfood scrambled eggs/tofu, finding those extra few minutes in the morning, will yield rewards not only for your day but for your weight and health over the longer term.

With Sirtfoods working to overcharge our energy levels, there's, even more, to gain from getting a hit from them early in the morning to start your day. This is done not only by eating a Sirtfood-rich meal but also by consuming the green juice, which we suggest you have either first thing in the morning — at least thirty minutes before a meal — or midmorning. We get plenty of accounts from our own clinical experience of people who drink their green juice first thing and don't feel hungry for a few hours afterwards. If this is the impact, it has on you, waiting a few hours before getting breakfast is perfectly fine. Only don't miss this one.

Alternatively, with a good meal, you can kick off your day, then wait two or three hours to get the green juice. Be flexible, and simply go for something that works for you.

Sirtfood Bites

When it comes to snacking, you should take it, or leave it. So much debate has been raised about whether eating regular, smaller meals is better for weight loss, or just sticking to three healthy meals a day. The fact is, that's just not important.

The way we've designed the maintenance menu for you means you're going to eat three well-balanced Sirtfood-rich meals a day, and you might not need a snack, either. But maybe you've been busy with working out or dashing with the kids, and you need something to tide you to the following meal. And if that "little thing" will give you a whammy of Sirtfood nutrients and delicious taste, then it's happy days. That's why we developed our "Sirtfood bites." These smart little treats are a truly guilt-free treat made entirely from sirtfoods: almonds, walnuts, chocolate, extra virgin olive oil, and turmeric. We recommend eating one, or a maximum of two, every day for the days that you need them.

"Sirtifying" Your Meals

We've noticed that inclusion, not exclusion is the only healthy diet. But true success goes beyond this — the diet has to be consistent with living in modern times. Whether it's the ease of meeting our hectic life's demands or fitting in with our position as the bon vivant at dinner parties, the way we eat should be trouble-free. You will enjoy your svelte body and radiant glow, rather than thinking about the demands and restrictions of kooky foods.

What makes Sirtfoods so fantastic is that they are very available, familiar, and easy to include in your diet. Here, as you cross the gap between step 1 and routine eating, you can lay the groundwork for a new, enhanced lifelong eating strategy.

The main idea is what we call your meals, "Sirtifying." This is where we take popular dishes, including several classic classics, and we keep all the great taste with some clever swaps and easy Sirtfood inclusions but add a lot of goodness to that. You'll see just how easily this is done during Phase 2.

Examples include our delicious smoothie Sirtfood for the perfect on-the-go breakfast in a time-consuming environment and the easy move from wheat to buckwheat to add extra flavor and zip to the much-loved pasta comfort food.

Meanwhile, classic, famous dishes such as chili con carne and curry don't even need much improvement, with Sirtfood bonanzas offering traditional recipes. And who has said that fast food means bad food? Once you make it yourself, we combine the authentic, vivid flavors of a pizza and remove the shame. There's no need to say goodbye to indulgence either, as our smothered pancakes with berries and dark chocolate sauce have proven. It's not even a dessert, it's breakfast, and for you it's perfect. Easy changes: you keep eating the foods that you enjoy when maintaining a healthy weight and wellbeing. And that is Sirtfoods, the dietary revolution.

Cooking for More

To support this, we are now entering a stage called "Sirtfoods for All," where the recipes begin to appeal to more than one mouth. Whether it's for family or friends, the new recipes for dinner, as well as the Sirtfood-packed soup that we introduce in this process, are planned with four in mind. And why not take advantage of cooking batch meals to freeze for those already cooking for one or two to have meals ready for the coming week?

Q&A

You should have found responses to most of your questions about the Sirt diet in the pages here.

However, I will try to find to answer any residual questions you might have so that you can begin your trip to success with more confidence.

Is Sirtfood healthy for children?

Children should avoid wine, coffee, and other highly caffeinated foods, such as Matcha. On the other hand, children can enjoy sirtuin-rich foods such as cabbage, eggplant, blueberries, and dates with their regular diet. Yet, while children can enjoy most sirtuin-rich foods, that is not the same as to say that they can practice the Sirt diet.

This diet plan is not intended for children, and it does not fit the needs of their growing bodies.

Practicing this diet plan could not only negatively affect them physically, but it could injury their mental health for years to come.
Anybody can develop an eating disorder, but it is particularly true for children.

If you want your child to eat healthily, ensure they eat a wide range of foods, as suggested by their doctor, and you can simply include plenty of sirtuin-rich foods into what they are already eating.

Put the focus on eating healthfully and not losing weight. Even if your child's doctor does want them to lose weight, you don't need to make the child aware of this fact. You can help guide them along with a healthy lifestyle, coaching them on how to eat well and stay active over sports and play, and the weight will come off naturally.

For similar reasons, you can include sirtfoods in a balanced diet while pregnant, but you should avoid an active Sirt diet when you are pregnant.

It doesn't contain the number of requirements for either a pregnant woman or a growing baby.

Save the diet for after you have delivered a healthy baby, and both you and your child will be healthy and happy.

Can I Exercise During Stage One?

If you are used to doing yoga and a spin class a few times a week, keep it up! If you are used to running a few miles a day, have at it! Do what you and your body are comfortable with, and as your doctor advises, and you should be fine

I'm Tinny. Can I Follow the Diet? Whether or not you can follow the first phase of the Sirt diet will depend just how thin you already are. While a person who is overweight or well within a healthy weight can practice the first phase, nobody who is clinically underweight should.

You can know if you are underweighting by calculating your Body Mass Index, or BMI. There are plenty of BMI calculators online, and if yours is at nineteen points or below, you should avoid the first stage of the diet.

It is always a good idea to ask your doctor if it is safe for you to lose weight, and if the Sirt diet is safe for your condition. While the Sirt diet is generally safe for people with certain illnesses, it may not be the case. While it is understandable to desire to be even more thin, even if you already are thin, pushing yourself past the point of being underweight is incredibly unhealthy, both physically and mentally.

Some of the side effects of force your body to extreme weight loss include bone loss and osteoporosis, lowered immune system, fertility problems, and an increased risk of heart disease.

If you want to benefit from the health of the Sirt diet and are underweight, assume the calories, your doctor recommends, along with plenty of sirtfoods.

This will ensure you preserve a healthy weight while also receiving the benefits that sirtuins have to offer.

If you are thin, but still at a BMI of twenty to twenty-five, then you should be safe beginning the Sirt diet, unless otherwise instructed by your doctor.

Can You Eat Meat and Dairy on The Sirtfood Diet?

In many recipes, we choose to use sirtfood sources of protein, such as soy, walnuts, and buckwheat.

This does not mean that you aren't allowed to enjoy meat on the Sirt diet.
It's easy to enjoy a vegetarian or vegan Sirt diet, but if you love your sources of meat, then you don't have to give them up.

Protein is an essential aspect of the Sirt diet to preserve muscle tone, and whether you consume only plant-based proteins or a mixture of plant and animal-based proteins is entirely up to you.

Some meats can help you well utilize the sirtfoods you eat because the amino acid leucine can enhance the effect of sirtfoods. You can find this amino acid in chicken, beef, pork, fish, eggs, dairy, and tofu.

Can I Drink Red Wine during Stage One?

As your calories will be so limited during the first phase, it is not advised to drink alcohol during this phase. Yet, you can enjoy it in moderation during stage two and the maintenance stage.

Chapter 15: Breakfast Recipes Sirtfood

Mushroom Scramble Eggs

Preparation Time: 10 minutes
Cooking Time: 10 minutes
Servings: 4

Ingredients:

- ✓ 2 tbsp
- ✓ 1 teaspoon ground garlic
- ✓ 1 teaspoon mild curry powder
- ✓ 20g lettuce, approximately sliced
- ✓ 1 teaspoon extra virgin olive oil
- ✓ 1/2 bird's eye peeled, thinly chopped
- ✓ a couple of mushrooms, finely chopped
- ✓ 5g parsley, finely chopped

*elective * Insert a seed mix for a topper plus Some Rooster Sauce for taste

Directions:

1. Mix the curry and garlic powder together and then add just a little water until a light glue is obtained.
2. Steam the lettuce for 2 to 3 minutes.
3. Heat the oil over moderate heat in a skillet, and fry the chili and mushrooms for 2 - 3 minutes until they begin to soften and brown.
4. Insert the eggs and spice paste and cook over moderate heat, then add the carrot and then proceed to cook over a moderate heat for a further minute. In the end, put in the parsley, mix well, and function.

Nutrition:

- ✓ Calories: 43 Cal
- ✓ Fat: 2.33 g
- ✓ Protein: 1.25 g
- ✓ Sugar: 0.39 g

Blue Hawaii Smoothie

Preparation Time: 5 minutes
Cooking Time: 0 minutes
Servings: 1

Ingredients:

- ✓ 2 tablespoons rings or approximately 4-5 balls
- ✓ 1/2 cup frozen tomatoes
- ✓ two Tbsp ground flaxseed
- ✓ ⅛ cup tender coconut (unsweetened, organic)
- ✓ few walnuts
- ✓ 1/2 cup fat-free yogurt
- ✓ 5-6 ice cubes
- ✓ dab of water

Directions:

Throw all of the ingredients together and combine until smooth. You might need to prevent and wake up to receive it combined smoothie or put in more water.

Nutrition:

- ✓ Calories: 222 Cal
- ✓ Fat: 12.53 g
- ✓ Protein: 12.91 g
- ✓ Sugar: 11.39 g

Turkey Breakfast Sausages

Preparation Time: 15 minutes
Cooking Time: 20 minutes
Servings: 2

Ingredients:

✓   1 lb. extra lean ground turkey
✓   1 Tbsp EVOO, and a little more to dirt pan
✓   1 Tbsp fennel seeds
✓   2 teaspoons smoked paprika
✓   1 teaspoon red pepper flakes
✓   1 teaspoon peppermint
✓   1 teaspoon chicken seasoning
✓   A couple of shredded cheddar cheese
✓   A couple of chives, finely chopped
✓   A few shakes garlic and onion powder
✓   Two spins of pepper and salt

Directions:

1. Pre Heat oven to 350F.
2. Utilize a little EVOO to dirt a miniature muffin pan.
3. Combine all ingredients and blend thoroughly.
4. Fill each pit on top of the pan and then cook for approximately 15-20 minutes. Each toaster differs; therefore, when muffin fever is 165, then remove.

Nutrition:

✓ Calories: 168 Cal
✓ Fat: 44.71 g
✓ Protein: 285.92 g
✓ Sugar: 3.71 g

Banana Pecan Muffins

Preparation Time: 20 minutes
Cooking Time: 40 minutes
Servings: 12

Ingredients:

- ✓ 3 Tbsp butter softened
- ✓ 4 ripe bananas
- ✓ 1 Tbsp honey
- ✓ ⅛ cup OJ
- ✓ 1 teaspoon cinnamon
- ✓ 2 cups all-purpose pasta
- ✓ 2 capsules
- ✓ a couple of pecans, sliced
- ✓ 1 Tbsp vanilla

Directions:

1. Preheat the oven to 180ºC.
2. Lightly oil the sides and bottom of the muffin tin and then dust with flour.
3. Dust the surfaces of the tin gently with flour then tap to eradicate any excess.
4. Peel and insert the batter to a mixing bowl and with a fork, mash the carrots; therefore, that you've got a combination of chunky and smooth, then put aside.
5. Insert the orange juice, melted butter, eggs, vanilla, and spices and stir to combine. Roughly chop the pecans onto a chopping board, when using, then fold throughout the mix. Spoon at the batter 3/4 full and bake in the oven for approximately 40 minutes, or until golden and cooked through.

Nutrition:

- ✓ Calories: 132 Cal
- ✓ Fat: 37.04 g
- ✓ Protein: 26.36 g
- ✓ Sugar: 19.65 g

Banana and Blueberry Muffins - SRC

Preparation Time: 20 minutes
Cooking Time: 30 minutes
Servings: 10

Ingredients:

✓ 4 large ripe bananas, peeled and mashed
✓ 3/4 cup of sugar
✓ 1 egg, lightly crushed
✓ 1/2 cup of butter, melted (and a little extra to dust the interiors of this muffin tin)
✓ 2 cups of blueberries (if they are suspended, do not Defrost them. simply pop them into the batter suspended and)
✓ 1 teaspoon baking powder
✓ 1 teaspoon baking soda
✓ 1/2 teaspoon salt
✓ 1 cup of coconut bread
✓ 1/2 cup of flour (or 1-1; two cup bread)
✓ 1/2 cup applesauce
✓ dab of cinnamon

Directions:

1. Add mashed banana to a large mixing bowl.
2. Insert sugar & egg and mix well.
3. Add peanut butter and strawberries.
4. Sift all the dry ingredients together, then add the dry ingredients into the wet mix and mix together lightly.
5. Set into 12 greased muffin cups
6. Bake for 20-30min in 180C or 350 F.

Nutrition:

✓ Calories: 203 Cal
✓ Fat: 106.48 g
✓ Protein: 21.8 g
✓ Sugar: 196 g

Morning Meal Sausage Gravy

Preparation Time: 5 minutes
Cooking Time: 5 minutes
Servings: 1

Ingredients:

✓ 1 lb. sausage
✓ 2 cups 2 percent milk (complete is great also)
✓ 1/4 cup entire wheat bread
✓ salt and a Lot of pepper to flavor

Directions:

1. Cook sausage from skillet.
2. Add flour and blend cook for about a minute.
3. Insert two cups of milk.
4. Whisk Whilst gravy thickens and bubbles.
5. Add pepper and salt and keep to taste until flawless.
6. Let stand a minute or so to ditch and function over several snacks.

Nutrition:

✓ Calories: 260 Cal
✓ Fat: 98.99 g
✓ Protein: 104.43 g
✓ Sugar: 27.05 g

Easy Egg-White Muffins

Preparation Time: 20 minutes
Cooking Time: 1 hour
Servings: 8

Ingredients:

- ✓ Language muffin - I enjoy Ezekiel 7 grain
- ✓ egg-whites - 6 tbsp or two large egg whites
- ✓ turkey bacon or bacon sausage
- ✓ sharp cheddar cheese or gouda
- ✓ green berry
- ✓ discretionary - lettuce, and hot sauce, hummus, flaxseeds, etc.

Directions:

1. At a microwavable safe container, then spray entirely to stop the egg from adhering, then pour egg whites into the dish.
2. Lay turkey bacon or bacon sausage paper towel and then cook.
3. Subsequently, toast your muffin, if preferred.
4. Then put the egg dish in the microwave for 30 minutes. Afterward, with a spoon or fork, then immediately flip egg within the dish and cook for another 30 minutes. Whilst dish remains hot sprinkle some cheese while preparing sausage.
5. The secret is to get a paste of some kind between each coating to put up the sandwich together, i.e., a very small little bit of hummus or even cheese.

Nutrition:

- ✓ Calories: 837 Cal
- ✓ Fat: 34.95 g
- ✓ Protein: 14.71 g
- ✓ Sugar: 68.61 g

Sweet Potato Hash

Preparation Time: 10 minutes
Cooking Time: 10 minutes
Servings: 4

Ingredients:

✓ Inch Sweet-potato
✓ 1/2 red pepper, diced
✓ 3 green onions, peppermint
✓ leftover turkey, then sliced into bits (optional)
✓ 1 Tbsp of butter - perhaps a bit less (I never quantify)
✓ carrot powder - a few shakes
✓ Pepper - only a small dab to get a bit of warmth
✓ pepper and salt to flavor
✓ scatter of cheddar cheese (optional)

Directions:

1. Stab a sweet potato and microwave for 5 minutes.
2. Remove from microwave, peel the skin off, and foliage.
3. At a skillet, on medium-high warmth, place peppers and butter and sauté to get a few minutes.
4. Insert potato bits and keep sautéing.
5. Whilst sauté, add sweeteners, leafy vegetables, and green onions.
6. Insert a dab of cheddar and Revel in!

Nutrition:

✓ Calories: 145 Cal
✓ Fat: 11.79 g
✓ Protein: 1.79 g
✓ Sugar: 5.08 g

Asparagus, Mushroom Artichoke Strata

Preparation Time: 20 minutes
Cooking Time: 15 minutes
Servings: 2

Ingredients:

- ✓ Inch little loaf of sourdough bread
- ✓ 4 challah rolls
- ✓ 8 eggs
- ✓ 2 cups of milk
- ✓ 1 teaspoon salt
- ✓ 1/4 teaspoon black pepper
- ✓ 1 cup Fontina cheese, cut into little chunks
- ✓ 1/2 cup shredded Parmesan cheese
- ✓ 1 Tbsp butter (I used jojoba)
- ✓ 1 teaspoon dried mustard
- ✓ 1/2 can of artichoke hearts, sliced
- ✓ 1 bunch green onions, grated
- ✓ 1 bunch asparagus, cut into 1-inch bits
- ✓ 1 10oz package of baby Bella (cremini) mushrooms, chopped

Directions:

1. Clean mushrooms and slice and trim asparagus and cut in 1-inch pieces. Reserve in a bowl and scatter 1/2 teaspoon salt mixture.
2. Drain and dice 1/2 may or modest artichoke hearts.
3. Melt butter in a pan over moderate heat, also sauté the asparagus and mushrooms before the mushrooms start to brown, about 10 minutes.
4. Blend the artichoke core pieces into a bowl with all a mushroom/asparagus mix. Set aside.
5. Cut or split a tiny sourdough loaf into 1-inch bits. (My loaf was a little too small, therefore that I used 4 challah rolls too)
6. Grease a 9x13 inch baking dish and generate a base coating of bread at the dish. Spread 1/2 cup of Fontina cheese bread, at a coating, and disperse half an apple mixture on the cheese. Lay-down a different layer of these vegetables and bread and high using a 1/2 cup of Fontina cheese.
7. Whisk together eggs, salt, milk, dry mustard, and pepper into a bowl and then pour the egg mixture on the vegetables and bread.
8. Cover the dish, and then simmer for 3 weeks.
9. Pre Heat oven to 375 degrees.
10. Eliminate the casserole from the fridge and let stand for half an hour.
11. Spread All the Parmesan cheese at a coating within the strata.
12. Bake in the preheated oven until a time when a knife inserted near the border comes out clean, 40 to 45 minutes. Allow it stand 5 to 10 minutes before cutting into squares.

Nutrition: (Calories: 350 Cal | Fat: 169 g | Protein: 181 g | Sugar: 49.76 g)

Egg White Veggie Wontons W/Fontina Topped W/ Crispy Prosciutto

Preparation Time: 15 minutes
Cooking Time: 15 minutes
Servings: 4

Ingredients:

- ✓ 1 cup egg whites
- ✓ butter
- ✓ fontina cheese
- ✓ mixed shredded cheddar cheese
- ✓ broccoli I utilized wheat, chopped bits
- ✓ tomatoes - diced
- ✓ salt and pepper
- ✓ prosciutto - two pieces
- ✓ Remove Won Ton wrappers out of the freezer.

Directions:

1. Pre Heat oven to 350.
2. Spray miniature cupcake tin with cooking spray.
3. After wrappers begin to defrost, peel off them carefully - apart, one at a time and press cupcake tin lightly.
4. I sliced the wrappers having a little bit of peanut butter. (optional)
5. set a chunk of cheese in every bottom.
6. Satisfy desired lettuce - I used pre-cooked broccoli bits and diced tomatoes.
7. Pour egg whites all toppings.
8. Sprinkle each with some of those shredded cheddar cheese.
9. Cook for approximately 15 minutes, but get started watching them afterward 10 - whenever they poof up - assess them poking the middle with a fork.
10. While eggs are cooking, then spray a sheet of foil with cooking spray and then put 2 pieces of prosciutto onto it and then cook at exactly the exact same period as the egg whites. After 8 minutes, then take and let sit once it cools it becomes crispy and chop and high eggs!

Nutrition:

- ✓ Calories: 298 Cal
- ✓ Fat: 11 g
- ✓ Protein: 24 g
- ✓ Sugar: 6 g

Chapter 16: Power Juice and Cocktail Recipes

Lemonade Redneck

Preparation Time: 5 minutes
Cooking Time: 5 minutes
Servings: 1

Ingredients:

- ✓ Bourbon
- ✓ Ice cubes
- ✓ Lemonade
- ✓ A slice of lemon

Directions:

1. Take your mason jar
2. Fill it with ice cubes
3. Pour bourbon
4. Add the lemonade
5. Slice a lemon
6. Add the slices to the pot
7. Serve (without straw, it's more authentic but it's less practical)

Nutrition:

- ✓ Calories: 11 Cal
- ✓ Fat: 0.12 g
- ✓ Protein: 0.17 g
- ✓ Sugar: 1.21 g

Coffee Latte Milkshake

Preparation Time: 2 minutes
Cooking Time: 2 minutes
Servings: 1

Ingredients:

- ✓ 350ml cold coffee (1 1/2 cups)
- ✓ 2 scoops of vanilla ice cream
- ✓ 2 tablespoons chocolate syrup or even better, Hot fudge
- ✓ Whipped cream
- ✓ Squares of "rich" dark chocolate - dessert type

Directions:

1. Take a blender
2. Pour coffee
3. Put the scoops of ice cream
4. Pour syrup
5. Mix well
6. Optional: pour some chocolate syrup coulis into the glass, tilting it diagonally, as if you were
7. pouring beer. It's super beautiful but be careful, you have to pour the milkshake gently after
8. Pour the milkshake into the glass
9. Cover with whipped cream
10. Chop the chocolate over the top and serve

Nutrition:

- ✓ Calories: 218 Cal
- ✓ Fat: 0.88 g
- ✓ Protein: 1.64 g
- ✓ Sugar: 38.73 g

Berry and Beet Smoothie

Preparation Time: 5 minutes
Cooking Time: 5 minutes
Servings: 1

Ingredients:

- ✓ 1 cup of pineapple juice
- ✓ 1 cup of low-fat or fat-free vanilla yogurt
- ✓ 1 cup of fresh or frozen strawberries
- ✓ 1/2 cup of fresh or frozen blueberries
- ✓ 1/2 cup of beet canned sliced, drained

Directions:

1. Combine all ingredients in a blender.
2. Mix until smooth.
3. Serve immediately.
4. Refrigerate or freeze what is leftover during the following 2 hours.

Notes : For a thicker smoothie, use frozen fruit instead of fresh fruit.

5. Use plain yogurt and ½ teaspoon of vanilla.
6. Add a banana.

Nutrition:

- ✓ Calories: 662 Cal
- ✓ Fat: 4.68 g
- ✓ Protein: 16.54 g
- ✓ Sugar: 123.81 g

Green Pineapple Smoothie

Preparation Time: 5 minutes
Cooking Time: 5 minutes
Servings: 1

Ingredients:

✓   50 grams of chard
✓   1 apple
✓   200 grams of pineapple
✓   1 tsp. of flax seeds

Directions:

All to the glass of the blender with a little water and grind well.

Nutrition:

✓ Calories: 251 Cal
✓ Fat: 4.11 g
✓ Protein: 7.3 g
✓ Sugar: 48.36 g

Blue Hawaii

The first Blue Hawaii was made by Harry Yee, the chief bartender at the Hilton Hawaiian Village Hotel in Waikiki. Yee had to create a blue cocktail when a representative from a well-known distillery demanded a drink with that hue, since he was promoting Curaçao. Although the combination of ingredients has evolved, Blue Hawaii maintains rum as a base drink and the classic umbrella as the garnish.

Preparation Time: 5 minutes
Cooking Time: 5 minutes
Servings: 1

Ingredients:
- ✓ 60 ml of rum
- ✓ 30 ml of blue Curaçao
- ✓ 30 ml of orange juice
- ✓ 60 ml of pineapple juice

Directions:
Mix all ingredients inside a cocktail shaker with ice and shake well for a few seconds. Garnish the glass using a slice of pineapple or orange and serve. It has no loss, but if you are one of those who prefers to trace the movements of an expert, here is an example. Remember, Blue Hawaii is ideal to consume before eating, on a terrace in the sun.

Nutrition:
- ✓ Calories: 413 Cal
- ✓ Fat: 10.75 g
- ✓ Protein: 57.12 g
- ✓ Sugar: 0 g

Daiquiri

Thinking of Daiquiri is thinking of the beach, palm trees, music, summer ... is thinking of Cuba. There is born this cocktail that is ordered in bars around the world and whose basic alcohol is white rum. The daiquiri owes its name to a beach near Santiago de Cuba and its origin to an American named Jennings Cox, who had to improvise a drink for his guests when he ran out of Geneva. And he mixed three

Preparation Time: 5 minutes
Cooking Time: 5 minutes
Servings: 1

Ingredients:

- ✓ 42 ml of white rum
- ✓ Juice of half a lemon (about 7 ml)
- ✓ 1 tablespoon of sugar

Directions:

The daiquiri was one of Ernest Hemingway's favorite drinks, that whenever he traveled to Cuba, he passed by La Floridita, a bar that claims to be the birthplace of the daiquiri and that hundreds of celebrities have visited since the American writer recommended it. So, if you want to have one of the best daiquiris in the world, stop by Havana. Although the original cocktail was made with lemon, it is easy to find strawberry, banana or assorted fruit daiquiris. Other variations lead us to the Floridita Daiquiri, which contains maraschino liqueur, or the Papa-Papa, in which the quantities are doubled and grapefruit is added.

Nutrition:

- ✓ Calories: 36 Cal
- ✓ Fat: 0.06 g
- ✓ Protein: 0.08 g
- ✓ Sugar: 8.43 g

Spinach Smoothie

Preparation Time: 5 minutes
Cooking Time: 5 minutes
Servings: 1

Ingredients:

- ✓ 1 large hand spinach (50 grams)
- ✓ 1 pear
- ✓ ½ banana
- ✓ ¼ zucchini
- ✓ 100 ml unsweetened almond milk
- ✓ 100 ml of water

Directions:

Get a blender; pour all the ingredients inside it, and then blend.

Nutrition:

- ✓ Calories: 1 Cal
- ✓ Fat: 0.01 g
- ✓ Protein: 0.08 g
- ✓ Sugar: 0 g

Kale Smoothie

Preparation Time: 5 minutes
Cooking Time: 5 minutes
Servings: 1

Ingredients:

✓   1 large hand kale (50 grams)
✓   ½ mango
✓   ½ banana
✓   1 tbsp chia seed
✓   100 ml unsweetened coconut milk
✓   150 ml of water

Directions:

Get a blender; pour all the ingredients into it, and then blend.

Nutrition:

✓ Calories: 290 Cal
✓ Fat: 15 g
✓ Protein: 68 g
✓ Sugar: 100 g

Avocado Smoothie

Preparation Time: 5 minutes
Cooking Time: 5 minutes
Servings: 1

Ingredients:

- ✓ ½ avocado
- ✓ 1 banana
- ✓ Hand of spinach
- ✓ 1 tbsp. linseed
- ✓ 100 ml unsweetened almond milk
- ✓ 100 ml of water

Directions:

Get a blender; pour all the ingredients into it, and then blend.

Nutrition:

- ✓ Calories: 161 Cal
- ✓ Fat: 14.73 g
- ✓ Protein: 2.01 g
- ✓ Sugar: 0.66 g

Lettuce Smoothie

Preparation Time: 5 minutes
Cooking Time: 5 minutes
Servings: 1

Ingredients:

- ✓ 2 hands turn
- ✓ 3 fresh plums, seeded
- ✓ ½ banana
- ✓ 1 tbsp. linseed
- ✓ ½ cucumbers
- ✓ 200 ml unsweetened almond milk

Directions:

Get a blender; pour all the ingredients into it, and then blend.

Nutrition:

- ✓ Calories: 135 Cal
- ✓ Fat: 0.3 g
- ✓ Protein: 1.09 g
- ✓ Sugar: 32.17 g

Chapter 17: Main Meal Recipes

Baked Potatoes with Spicy Chickpea Stew Fillet Diablo

Preparation Time: 10 minutes
Cooking Time: 15 minutes
Servings: 2

Ingredients:

- ✓ 2 fillets of sole (5 ounces each)
- ✓ 1 teaspoon lemon juice
- ✓ 1/2 teaspoon salt
- ✓ Garnish
- ✓ 2 thin lemon slices, chopped fresh parsley, and parsley sprigs
- ✓ 2 teaspoons margarine
- ✓ 1 teaspoon all-purpose flour
- ✓ 1/4 cup water
- ✓ 2 tablespoons dry white wine
- ✓ 1 teaspoon Dijon-style mustard
- ✓ 1 teaspoon drained capers
- ✓ 1/2 teaspoon grated lemon rind
- ✓ 1/2 teaspoon white pepper, divided

Directions:

In small saucepan heat margarine until bubbly and hot. Sprinkle with flour and stir quickly to combine; cook over low heat, constantly stirring, for 1 minute. Remove from heat; stir in water, wine, and mustard. Return to heat and bring mixture to a boil; reduce heat and let simmer, constantly stirring, until sauce is thickened. Stir in capers, lemon rind, and dash pepper; remove from heat and keep warm.

Sprinkle sole fillets with lemon juice and remaining pepper. Spray rack of broiling pan with nonstick cooking spray; transfer fish to rack and broil until fish flakes easily when tested with a fork, about 5 minutes. Sprinkle fillets with salt, then transfer to a serving platter. Spoon sauce over fish; garnish with lemon and parsley.

Nutrition:

- ✓ Calories: 167 Cal
- ✓ Fat: 5 g
- ✓ Protein: 24 g
- ✓ Sugar: 4.14 g

Artichoke-Stuffed Red Snapper

Preparation Time: 40 minutes
Cooking Time: 50 minutes
Servings: 6

Ingredients:

- ✓ 1 tablespoon vegetable oil
- ✓ 3/4 cup finely chopped onions
- ✓ 1/2 cups frozen artichoke hearts, thawed and chopped
- ✓ 3 slices white bread, toasted and made into fine crumbs
- ✓ 1/4 cup each chopped fresh parsley and lemon juice
- ✓ 1 teaspoon salt
- ✓ 1/2 teaspoon pepper
- ✓ 1 red snapper,
- ✓ 3 pounds dressed with head and tail left on 1 cup mixed vegetable juice

Directions:

Preheat oven to 350°F. In 9-inch skillet heat oil; add onions and sauté until translucent. Add artichoke hearts and sauté for 3 minutes longer. Stir in bread crumbs, parsley, lemon juice, salt, and pepper; remove from heat and allow the mixture to cool slightly.

Stuff fish with artichoke mixture, using toothpicks or wooden skewers to close the cavity. Spray baking dish that is large enough to hold fish flat with nonstick cooking spray; transfer stuffed snapper to a dish and pour vegetable juice over fish. Bake, frequently basting with pan juices, until fish flakes easily at the touch of a fork, 40 to 50 minutes.

Nutrition:

- ✓ Calories: 218 Cal
- ✓ Fat: 13 g
- ✓ Protein: 31 g
- ✓ Sugar: 11.25 g

Sesame Chicken Salad

Preparation Time: 10 minutes
Cooking Time: 12 minutes
Servings: 2

Ingredients:

✓   1 tbsp sesame seeds
✓   One cucumber, peeled, half-long, desired with a teaspoon and 100 g sliced baby kale, roughly chopped
✓   60 g Pak choi, very finely shredded
✓   1/2 red onion, very finely sliced
✓   A big handful (20 g) of petroleum, chopped
✓   150 g cooked chicken, shredded
✓   For dressing:
✓   1 tbsp of extra virgin olive oil
✓   1 tsp of sesame oil
✓   One lime juice
✓   1 tsp of sugar
✓   2 tsp of soy sauce

Directions:

1. In A hot frying pan, the sesame seeds toast for 2 minutes until lightly browned and fragrant.
2. Move to a cold plate.
3. Combine the olive oil, sesame oil, lime juice, honey, and soy sauce in a small bowl to make a dressing.
4. In a large bowl, put the cucumber, the kale, the Pak choi, the red onion, and the parsley and combine gently. Pour over the sauce, then again blend.
5. Divide the salad with the shredded chicken between two plates, and top. Just before eating, brush over the sesame seeds.

Nutrition:

✓ Calories: 304 Cal
✓ Fat: 95.86 g
✓ Protein: 74.38 g
✓ Sugar: 6.37 g

Sirt Food Miso-Marinated Cod with Stir-Fried Greens

Preparation Time: 10 minutes
Cooking Time: 10 minutes
Servings: 2

Ingredients:

- ✓ 20g miso
- ✓ 1 tbsp mirin
- ✓ 1 tbsp of extra virgin olive oil
- ✓ 200 g of skinless cod fillet
- ✓ 20 g of red onion, sliced
- ✓ 40 g of celery, sliced
- ✓ One garlic clove, finely chopped
- ✓ One bird's eye chili, finely chopped
- ✓ 1 tsp of fresh ginger
- ✓ 60 g of green beans
- ✓ 50 g of kale, roughly chopped
- ✓ 1 tsp of sesame seeds
- ✓ 5 g of parsley, roughly chopped
- ✓ 1 tbsp of tamari
- ✓ 30 g of buckwheat
- ✓ 1 tsp of turmeric

Directions:

Mix the miso, mirin, and oil in a tablespoon. Rub the cod all over and leave for 30 minutes to marinate. Bake the cod for about 10 minutes.

Meanwhile, heat the remaining oil to a large frying pan or wok. Stir-fry the onion for a few minutes, then add the celery, garlic, chili, ginger, green beans, and kale. Toss and fry until the kale is cooked through and tender. To aid the cooking process, you might need to add a little water to the pan. Cook the buckwheat with the turmeric for 3 minutes according to the directions on the packet. To the stir-fry, add the sesame seeds, parsley, and tamari and serve with the greens and fish.

Nutrition:

- ✓ Calories: 355 Cal
- ✓ Fat: 10.87 g
- ✓ Protein: 40.31 g
- ✓ Sugar: 5.17 g

Raspberry and Blackcurrant Jelly-Sirtfood Recipes

Preparation Time: 15 minutes
Cooking Time: 15 minutes plus setting time
Servings: 3

Ingredients:

✓   100g raspberries washed
✓   Two leaves
✓   100g blackcurrants washed and stalked removed
✓   2 tbsp granulated sugar
✓   300ml water

Directions:

1. Two of your SIRT 5 a day, making a jelly ahead of time, is a perfect way to prepare the fruit, so it's ready to eat the first morning.
2. Put the raspberries in two plates/glasses/molds. Place the gelatin leaves softening in a bowl of cold water.
3. Put the blackcurrants with the sugar and 100ml water in a small saucepan and bring to a boil.
4. Simmer hard for 5 minutes, then remove from heat. Put on for 2 minutes.

5. Squeeze the gelatin leaves out of the excess water and add to the saucepan. Remove until completely dissolved, and then mix in the remaining water. The jellies should be ready overnight or in around 3-4 hours.

Nutrition:

✓ Calories: 142 Cal
✓ Fat: 1 g
✓ Protein: 4.18 g
✓ Sugar: 20.07 g

Strawberry Buckwheat Tabouleh

Preparation Time: 15 minutes
Cooking Time: 15 minutes
Servings: 4

Ingredients:

- ✓ 50 g of buckwheat
- ✓ 1 tbsp of turmeric
- ✓ 80 g of avocado
- ✓ 65 g of tomato
- ✓ 20 g of red onion
- ✓ 25 g of Medjool dates, pitted
- ✓ 1 tbsp seed, 30 g of parsley
- ✓ 100 g of strawberries, hulled
- ✓ 1 tbsp of extra virgin olive oil
- ✓ 1/2 lemon juice, 30 g of rocket

Directions:

Cook the buckwheat with the turmeric, as indicated on the packet. Drain to cool and hold to one side. Cut the avocado, tomato, red onion, eggs, capers, and peregrinate thinly and blend with the cold buckwheat. Slice the strawberries, then mix the oil and lemon juice gently into the salad. Serve on a bed of rocket.

Nutrition:

- ✓ Calories: 382 Cal
- ✓ Fat: 19.34 g
- ✓ Protein: 6.5 g
- ✓ Sugar: 23.84 g

Buckwheat and Nut Loaf

Preparation Time: 15 minutes
Cooking Time: 15 minutes
Servings: 4

Ingredients:

✓   225g/8 oz. buckwheat
✓   2 tbsp olive oil
✓   225g/8 of mushrooms
✓   2-3 carrots, finely diced
✓   2-3 tbsp of fresh herbs, finely chopped
✓   225g/8 of nuts, e.g., hazelnuts, almonds, walnuts
✓   Two eggs, beaten (or 2 tbsp tahini for vegan version), salt and pepper

Directions:

Place the buckwheat in a 350 ml/1,5 cup pan with water and a pinch of salt. Take to simmer. Cover and cook with the lid until all the water is absorbed about 10-15 minutes. Blitz, the food processor's nuts, until well chopped.

Stir in the eggs and mix the potatoes, cooked buckwheat, herbs, and chopped nuts. If you use tahini instead of eggs, combine this with some water before combining it in the buckwheat to create a thick consistency of pouring. Switch to a lined or oiled loaf tin and bake for 30 minutes in the oven at gas mark 5/190C until set and just brown on top.

Nutrition:

✓ Calories: 279 Cal
✓ Fat: 19.1 g
✓ Protein: 69.8 g
✓ Sugar: 19.69 g

Moong Dahl

Preparation Time: 10 minutes
Cooking Time: 15 minutes
Servings: 5

Ingredients:

- ✓ 300g/10 of split mung beans (Moong Dahl)–preferably soaked for a few hours
- ✓ 600ml/1pt water
- ✓ Two tbsp/30 g olive oil, butter or ghee
- ✓ One red onion, finely chopped
- ✓ 1-2 tsp of coriander seeds
- ✓ 1-2 tsp of cumin seeds
- ✓ 2-4 tsp of fresh ginger, chopped
- ✓ 1-2 tsp of turmeric
- ✓ 1/4 tsp of cayenne pepper–more if you want it spicy
- ✓ Salt & black pepper to taste

Directions:

1. Drain and rinse split mung beans. Place in a casserole, and cover with water. Bring to the boil and skim off any moisture that comes up. Turn the heat down, cover and simmer.
2. In a heavy-bottomed pan, dry fry the coriander and cumin seeds until they begin to pop. Grind them in a mortar and pestle.
3. Attach the ground spices and the ginger, turmeric, and cayenne pepper to the onions. Cook in a couple of minutes.

Nutrition:

- ✓ Calories: 430 Cal
- ✓ Fat: 32.1 g
- ✓ Protein: 12.37 g
- ✓ Sugar: 17.3 g

Polenta Bake

Preparation Time: 20 minutes
Cooking Time: 50 minutes
Servings: 10

Ingredients:

- ✓ 850ml/1.5 pints of water
- ✓ 1 tsp of rock salt or sea salt
- ✓ 200g/7 of coarse yellow polenta
- ✓ 2 tsp of dried oregano
- ✓ 1 cup of sun-dried tomatoes
- ✓ Chopped, three eggs, separated
- ✓ 1-2 tbsp of butter or olive oil
- ✓ Freshly ground black pepper
- ✓ 300g/10 of cheddar or red Leicester cheese rubbed (optional)

Directions:

1. To cook the polenta, bring the water to a boil in a large salt pan.
2. Slowly pour in the boiling polenta the whole time. Remove the sun-dried tomatoes and the oregano.
3. Cook on low heat, as long as the polenta packet instructions suggest. It could be from 3 minutes to 40 minutes at any location. Remove to prevent clumping and to stick on frequently. Whereas the polenta cooks whip the egg whites until they form steep peaks.
4. When cooking the polenta, turn off the heat and mix egg yolks and black pepper in 1-2 tbsp of butter or olive oil together with 2/3 of the cheese, if used. Carefully insert the egg whites into the polenta mix.
5. Move the mixture to an evidence dish oiled with an oven: spread and the top smooth.
6. Sprinkle over the remaining grated cheese.
7. Bake for 40-50 minutes at gas mark 4/180C/350F, until set and start to brown.

Nutrition:

- ✓ Calories: 234 Cal
- ✓ Fat: 135.39 g
- ✓ Protein: 102.98 g
- ✓ Sugar: 25.37 g

Cajun Steak and Veg Rice Jar Recipe

Preparation Time: 15 minutes
Cooking Time: 20 minutes
Servings: 1

Ingredients:

✓ 1 tablespoon vegetable oil
✓ 1 celery stick, finely chopped
✓ 3 large carrots, sliced into rounds
✓ 250g frozen chopped mixed peppers
✓ 4 spring onions, chopped, green and white parts split
✓ 500g 5 percent beef mince
✓ 2 teaspoon seasoning
✓ 1 teaspoon tomato purée
✓ 2 x 250g packs ready-cooked long-grain rice

Directions:

1. Heat the oil in a large, shallow skillet over moderate heat. Add the carrots, celery, peppers, and snowy areas of the nuts. Cook for 10 mins before the veg is beginning to soften.
2. Insert the mince, season liberally, and cook for 10 mins before mince is browned and start to really go crispy.
3. Insert the Cajun seasoning and tomato purée; stir fry to coat the mince. Hint inside the rice combined with 4 tablespoons of plain water. Stir to completely unite heat and heat until the rice is hot. Scatter on the rest of the spring onion before serving.

Nutrition:

✓ Calories: 398 Cal
✓ Fat: 96.64 g
✓ Protein: 135.12 g
✓ Sugar: 16.8 g

Chapter Eighteen: Stir Fry Recipes

Chicken and Green Beans

Preparation Time: 6 minutes
Cooking Time: 10 minutes
Servings: 4

Ingredients:
- ✓ Toasted peanuts, for sprinkling
- ✓ For the Marinade:
- ✓ 1½ teaspoons cornstarch
- ✓ ½ teaspoon red pepper flakes, or to taste
- ✓ Salt, to taste
- ✓ 1 tablespoon soy sauce

For the Sauce:
- ✓ 2 tablespoons soy sauce, divided
- ✓ 2 tablespoons seasoned rice vinegar
- ✓ 2 tablespoons Chinese cooking wine
- ✓ 1-pound chicken thighs or breasts, boneless, skinless, sliced thinly against the grain
- ✓ 2 tablespoons of vegetable oil, broken down
- ✓ 6 Scallions, trimmed ends, cut into 1 "pieces
- ✓ 1 (2-inch) piece of ginger, sliced
- ✓ ¾ pound green beans, trimmed and halved
- ✓ Salt, to taste

Directions:
1. Combine marinade ingredients in a bowl, add chicken slices and toss.
2. In a small bowl, stir sauce ingredients together. Set aside.
3. In a wok, skillet, or frying pan, heat 1 tablespoon oil to shimmering.
4. Add Ginger and Scallion. Stir-fry until brown (roughly 2 minutes).
5. Add green beans and a pinch of salt, tossing until crisp-tender (about 4 minutes). Transfer
6. veggies to a platter and keep the wok warm.
7. Add remaining oil and adjust heat to high.
8. When the oil is almost smoking, lay the chicken on the wok and let cook until underside is
9. browned (about 1 minute).
10. Stir-fry for 1–2 minutes, or until evenly browned.
11. Stir in sauce and veggies.
12. Toss until sauce is thickened (about 30 seconds).
13. Remove from heat and season with more salt, if needed.
14. Sprinkle with toasted nuts and serve with rice.

***Nutrition:** (Calories: 563 Cal | Fat: 35 g | Protein: 84 g | Sugar: 13 g)*

Moo Goo Gai Pan (Mushrooms with Chicken)

Preparation Time: 5 minutes (add 15 minutes marinating time)
Cooking Time: 10 minutes
Servings: 2 - 4

Ingredients:

- ✓ ¾ pound chicken breasts, boneless and skinless, sliced thinly
- ✓ 3 tablespoons vegetable oil, divided
- ✓ 1 cup fresh button mushrooms, sliced
- ✓ ½ cup canned bamboo shoots, rinsed and drained
- ✓ ½ cup canned water chestnuts, rinsed and drained
- ✓ 1 thumb ginger, chopped
- ✓ 1 clove garlic, minced

For the Marinade:

- ✓ 2 tablespoons soy sauce
- ✓ 1 tablespoon Chinese cooking wine
- ✓ ½ teaspoon sesame oil, or to taste
- ✓ 1 tablespoon cornstarch

For the Sauce:

- ✓ ½ cup chicken stock or broth
- ✓ 2 tablespoons oyster sauce
- ✓ 1 teaspoon sugar
- ✓ 1 tablespoon cornstarch

Directions:

1. Combine ingredients for the marinade in a bowl with chicken. Rub into chicken and let marinate for 15 minutes.
2. In a bowl, mix sauce ingredients together and set aside.
3. In a wok, skillet, or frying pan, heat 2 tablespoons of oil.
4. Add the chicken to the surface and stir-fry until browned (about 3–5 minutes). Transfer onto a platform.
5. Add remaining oil to wok and stir-fry ginger and garlic until fragrant (about 30 seconds).
6. Stir in mushrooms and stir-fry for about 1 minute.
7. Add bamboo shoots and water chestnuts, stir-frying to heat through.
8. Give reserved sauce mixture a quick stir and pour into wok.
9. Cook, with stirring, until thickened.
10. Return chicken to wok and stir until well-coated and cooked through.

Nutrition: (Calories: 416 Cal | Fat: 15 g |Protein: 24 g | Sugar: 11.65 g)

Garlic Chicken

Preparation Time: 5 minutes
Cooking Time: 15 minutes
Servings: 4

Ingredients:

- ✓ 1½ Tablespoons of vegetable oil, broken down
- ✓ 1 pound of skinless, bare chicken breast cut into pieces of bite-size
- ✓ Salt and pepper to taste
- ✓ 1 cup broccoli florets
- ✓ 1 cup mushrooms, halved
- ✓ 1 yellow bell pepper, sliced thinly
- ✓ 4 cloves garlic, minced
- ✓ For the Sauce:
- ✓ ¾ cup chicken broth
- ✓ 1½ teaspoons sugar
- ✓ 1 tablespoon soy sauce
- ✓ 2 teaspoons sesame oil
- ✓ 2 teaspoons cornstarch

Directions:

1. In a bowl, stir ingredients of the sauce together and set aside.
2. Heat 1 spoonful of oil over high heat in a wok, skillet, or frying pan.
3. Add chicken, and add salt and pepper to season.
4. Stir-fry until browned on the surface (about 7 minutes). Transfer to a plate.
5. Add remaining oil to wok and heat over medium-high heat.
6. Add the broccoli, mushrooms, and bell pepper and stir-fry until tender (about 5 minutes).
7. Reduce heat to medium.
8. Add the garlic and stir-fry (about 30 seconds) until fragrant.
9. Back to wok chicken.
10. Give a quick stir to prepared sauce mixture and pour it into a wok.
11. Bring sauce to a boil and let simmer until thickened (about 2 minutes). Adjust flavor with more
12. salt and pepper, if needed.
13. Serve hot.

Nutrition: (Calories: 215 Cal | Fat: 6.3 g | Protein: 24 g | Sugar: 11.26 g)

Cashew Chicken

Preparation Time: 5 minutes plus 20 minutes marinating time
Cooking Time: 10 minutes
Servings: 3 - 4

Ingredients:

✓ 1-pound boneless, skinless chicken breasts, cubed
✓ 3–4 tablespoons oil for stir-frying, divided
✓ 1 clove garlic, minced
✓ 1 tablespoon green onion, chopped
✓ ¼ cup roasted cashew nuts

For the Marinade:

✓ 1 tablespoon Chinese cooking wine
✓ 2 teaspoons freshly squeezed ginger juice
✓ ½ teaspoon salt
✓ 1 tablespoon cornstarch

For the Sauce:

✓ 2 tablespoons hoisin sauce
✓ 2 tablespoons dark soy sauce
✓ 2 tablespoons water
✓ 1 teaspoon granulated sugar

Directions:

1. Combine the first 3 marinade ingredients and add chicken. Sprinkle with cornstarch and rub to coat. Let marinate for 20 minutes.
2. Stir sauce ingredients together in a bowl and set aside.
3. Heat 2 tablespoons oil in a wok, skillet, or frying pan over medium-high heat.
4. Add garlic and stir-fry until fragrant (about 30 seconds).
5. Add chicken and stir-fry until browned on the outside (about 5–7 minutes). Transfer to a plate.
6. Add remaining oil (about 1–2 tablespoons, or as needed) to wok.
7. Add green onion and stir-fry until tender.
8. Return chicken to wok and stir just to heat through.
9. Add sauce ingredients and cook until thickened.
10. Add cashews and stir until ingredients are well-coated with sauce.
11. Serve hot.

Nutrition: Calories: 396 Cal | Fat: 19 g | Protein: 34 g | Sugar: 43.62 g

Creamy Curry Chicken with Vegetables

Preparation Time: 25 minutes
Cooking Time: 15 minutes
Servings: 4

Ingredients:

✓ 1-pound boneless chicken breasts, cubed into small pieces
✓ 4 tablespoons green curry paste
✓ 1 cup reduced-fat coconut milk
✓ ½ cup chicken stock
✓ 2 zucchinis, sliced thinly
✓ 1 onion, diced
✓ 2 Asian eggplant (long and thin), sliced thinly
✓ 1 cup of broccoli, chopped into florets
✓ 2 tablespoons fresh basil
✓ ¼ teaspoon cayenne pepper, more if you like it spicier
✓ 1 teaspoon curry powder
✓ 2 tablespoons grapeseed oil
✓ 2 cups cooked brown or white rice for serving (optional)

Directions:

1. Heat oil on medium-high heat. When hot, add onion and curry paste and cook for 2 minutes.
2. Add chicken and stir-fry for 4-5 minutes. Be sure to coat it in the curry paste.
3. Add coconut milk and stock and bring to a boil. Turn down the heat to medium-low and let simmer for a few minutes.
4. Add the rest of the vegetables and the spices and cook until chicken is tender.
5. Serve over rice, if desired.

Nutrition:

✓ Calories: 300 Cal
✓ Fat: 11 g
✓ Protein: 28 g
✓ Sugar: 56.36 g

Simple Beef Stir-fry

Preparation Time: 15 minutes
Cooking Time: 25 minutes
Servings: 4

Ingredients:

✓   2 cups vegetable stock
✓   2 tablespoons soy sauce
✓   4 garlic cloves, chopped
✓   2 teaspoons chili powder
✓   1-pound top sirloin beef, thinly sliced
✓   3 cups broccoli, chopped into florets
✓   1 cup cremini mushrooms, sliced
✓   1 cup sugar snaps peas
✓   4 green onions, sliced
✓   1 tablespoon fresh ginger, peeled and sliced
✓   2 tablespoons grapeseed oil

Directions:

1. Prepare the marinade in a shallow dish or a re-sealable plastic bag such as a Zip-lock bag, Mix vegetable stock, soy sauce, and chili powder. If you desire more spices, add ½ teaspoon cayenne pepper. Toss the beef in the sauce and marinate for 10-15 minutes.
2. On high heat, add oil to the wok and when hot, put in ginger, broccoli, mushrooms, peas, green onions, and ¼ of the marinade, cook for about 3 minutes or until the broccoli softens. Add beef and remaining marinade and cook until beef is browned. Serve hot.

Nutrition:

✓ Calories: 390 Cal
✓ Fat: 21 g
✓ Protein: 30 g
✓ Sugar: 26 g

Easy Shiitake Stir-fry

Preparation Time: 2 minutes
Cooking Time: 7 – 10 minutes
Servings: 2

Ingredients:

✓ 2 tablespoons peanut oil
✓ 1 (½-inch) piece ginger, peeled and minced
✓ 1 clove garlic, minced
✓ ½ pound fresh shiitake mushrooms, sliced
✓ 1–2 tablespoons soy sauce
✓ 1 tablespoon sesame oil
✓ 1 green onion, chopped
✓ 2 teaspoons toasted sesame seeds

Directions:

1. Heat peanut oil in a wok, skillet, or frying pan over medium-high heat.
2. Stir-fry ginger and garlic until fragrant (about 30 seconds).
3. Add sliced shiitake and stir-fry until soft and lightly browned (about 2–3 minutes).
4. Stir in soy sauce and sesame oil.
5. Continue to stir-fry until most liquid has evaporated.
6. Sprinkle with green onion and sesame seeds.
7. Serve.

Nutrition:

✓ Calories: 283 Cal
✓ Fat: 22.9 g
✓ Protein: 3.8 g
✓ Sugar: 19.7 g

Okra Stir-fry

Preparation Time: 5 minutes
Cooking Time: 5 minutes
Servings: 2

Ingredients:

✓ 1 tablespoon peanut or vegetable oil
✓ 1 teaspoon Sichuan peppercorn
✓ 2 dried chili peppers, chopped
✓ 7 ounces okra, cut into bite-size pieces
✓ 2 teaspoons light soy sauce

Directions:

1. Heat oil in a wok, skillet, or frying pan over medium heat. Stir-fry Sichuan peppercorn until dark and fragrant (about 1 minute). Fish out the peppercorns and discard.
2. Add chili and stir-fry briefly (about 30 seconds).
3. Adjust heat to high.
4. Add okra and stir-fry to blanch and coat with oil (1 minute).
5. Add soy sauce. Reduce heat, if needed.
6. Continue stir-frying until okra is cooked through (about 3 minutes).
7. Serve hot.

Nutrition:

✓ Calories: 100 Cal
✓ Fat: 7 g
✓ Protein: 2.4 g
✓ Sugar: 8.9 g

Simple Stir-Fried Bok Choy

Preparation Time: 5 minutes
Cooking Time: 10 minutes
Servings: 4

Ingredients:

- ✓   1½ pounds bok choy, trimmed and washed
- ✓   2 tablespoons cooking oil
- ✓   2 cloves garlic, finely minced
- ✓   1 teaspoon grated ginger
- ✓   3 tablespoons water, broth or cooking wine
- ✓   1 teaspoon soy sauce
- ✓   ½ teaspoon sesame oil

Directions:

1. Add oil to wok, skillet, or frying pan.
2. Add garlic and ginger before the oil has been heated (this is to avoid burning the aromatics and
3. to infuse more flavor into the oil).
4. Set heat at medium-high.
5. Stir-fry when sizzling starts.
6. When fragrant and oil is adequately hot, stir in bok choy. Stir-fry to coat well with flavored oil and to cook evenly, until leaves turn bright green (about 15–30 seconds).
7. Splash with water, cover, and let steam for 1 minute.
8. Stir in soy sauce.
9. Remove from heat.
10. Drizzle with sesame oil and serve hot.

Nutrition:

- ✓ Calories: 91 Cal
- ✓ Fat: 11 g
- ✓ Protein: 2 g
- ✓ Sugar: 4 g

Lettuce Stir-fry

Preparation Time: 2 minutes
Cooking Time: 5 minutes
Servings: 4 - 6

Ingredients:

✓ 1½ teaspoons soy sauce
✓ 1½ teaspoons sesame oil
✓ 1 teaspoon of rice wine
✓ ¾ teaspoon sugar
✓ 1 tablespoon peanut or canola oil
✓ 3 cloves garlic, peeled and minced
✓ 1 head iceberg lettuce, rinsed, dried, and torn into large pieces
✓ Salt and pepper, to taste

Directions:

1. In a small bowl, stir together soy sauce, sesame oil, rice wine, and sugar. Set aside.
2. Heat oil in a wok, skillet, or frying pan over medium-high heat.
3. Stir-fry garlic until lightly browned.
4. Add lettuce and stir-fry very briefly until bright in color but still crisp.
5. Stir in sauce and season with salt and pepper.
6. Serve immediately.

Nutrition:

✓ Calories: 72 Cal
✓ Fat: 5.3 g
✓ Protein: 1.6 g
✓ Sugar: 5.7 g

Chapter 19: Sweets

Dark Chocolate Mousse (Vegan)

Preparation Time: 10 minutes
Cooking Time: 2 hours plus cooling time
Servings: 4

Ingredients:
- ✓ 1 (16 ounce) package silken tofu, drained
- ✓ ½ cup pure maple syrup
- ✓ 1 teaspoon pure vanilla extract
- ✓ ¼ cup soymilk
- ✓ ½ cup unsweetened cocoa powder
- ✓ Mint leaves (optional and highly encouraged)

Directions:
1. Place tofu, maple syrup and vanilla in a food processor or blender. Process until well blended.
2. Add remaining ingredients and process until mixture is fully blended.
3. Pour into small dessert cups or espresso cups. Chill for at least 2 hours.

Nutrition:
- ✓ Calories: 544 Cal
- ✓ Fat: 6.95 g
- ✓ Protein: 8.82 g
- ✓ Sugar: 99.75 g

Loaded Chocolate Fudge

Preparation Time: 10 minutes
Cooking Time: 1 hour plus cooling time
Servings: 16

Ingredients:

- ✓ 1 cup Medjool dates, chopped
- ✓ 2 tablespoons coconut oil, melted
- ✓ 1/2 cup peanut butter
- ✓ ¼ cup of unsweetened cocoa powder
- ✓ ½ cup walnuts
- ✓ 1 teaspoon vanilla

Directions:

1. Soak the dates in warm water for 20 – 30 minutes Lightly grease an 8" square baking pan with coconut oil.
2. Add dates, peanut butter, cocoa powder and vanilla to a food processer and blend until smooth.
3. Fold in walnuts.
4. Pack into the greased baking pan and put in your freezer for 1 hour or until fudge is solid and firm.
5. Cut into 16 or more bite-sized squares and store in a semi-airtight container in the refrigerator.

Nutrition:

- ✓ Calories: 992 Cal
- ✓ Fat: 79.21 g
- ✓ Protein: 19.51 g
- ✓ Sugar: 42.49 g

Chocolate Maple Walnuts

This is a super simple recipe that makes a great dinner party dessert that everyone can indulge in as much or as little as they personally choose. The maple syrup plays off the bitterness of the dark chocolate perfectly, and the walnuts provide just the right texture for your guests or family to sink their teeth into.

Preparation Time: 15 minutes
Cooking Time: 30 minutes
Servings: 2 cups od candied walnuts

Ingredients:

- ½ cup pure maple syrup, divided
- 2 cups raw, whole walnuts
- 5 squares of dark chocolate, at least 85%
- 1 ½ tablespoons coconut oil, melted
- 1 tablespoonful of water
- Sifted icing sugar
- 1 teaspoonful of vanilla extract

Directions:

1. Line a large baking sheet with parchment paper.
2. In a medium to large skillet, combine the walnuts and ¼ cup of maple syrup and cook over medium heat, stirring continuously, until walnuts are completely covered with syrup and golden in color, about 3 – 5 minutes.
3. Pour the walnuts onto the parchment paper and separate into individual pieces with a fork. Allow cooling completely, at least 15 minutes.
4. In the meantime, melt the chocolate in a double boiler with the coconut oil. Add the remaining maple syrup and stir until thoroughly combined.
5. When walnuts are cooled, transfer them to a glass bowl and pour the melted chocolate syrup over top. Use a silicone spatula to gently mix until walnuts are completely covered.
6. Transfer back to the parchment paper-lined baking sheet and, once again, separate each of the nuts with a fork.
7. Place the nuts in the fridge for 10 minutes or the freezer for 3 – 5 minutes, until chocolate has completely set.
8. Store in an airtight bag in your fridge.

Nutrition: Calories: 2033 Cal | Fat: 124.83 g | Protein: 24.43 g | Sugar: 197.74 g

Matcha and Chocolate Dipped Strawberries

Chocolate dipped strawberries are possibly one of the most romantic desserts of all time. They're also great for warm summer evenings when you're craving something sweet but don't want a heavy cake or pudding. Eating them any other evening of the year is also just right. You can't go wrong.

Preparation Time: 25 minutes
Cooking Time: 25 minutes
Servings: 4 - 6

Ingredients:
- 4 tablespoons cocoa butter
- 4 squares of dark chocolate, at least 85%
- ¼ cup of coconut oil
- 1 teaspoon Matcha green tea powder
- 20 – 25 large whole strawberries, stems on

Directions:
1. Melt cocoa butter, dark chocolate, coconut oil, and Matcha in a double boiler until nearly smooth.
2. Remove from heat and continue stirring until chocolate is completely melted.
3. Pour into a large glass bowl and stir constantly until the chocolate thickens and starts to lose its sheen, about 2 - 5 minutes.
4. Working one at a time, hold the strawberries by stems and dip into chocolate matcha mixture to coat. Let excess drip back into the bowl.
5. Place on a parchment-lined baking sheet and chill dipped berries in the fridge until the shell is set, 20–25 minutes.
6. You may need to reheat matcha mixture if it starts to set before you have dipped all the berries.

Nutrition:
- Calories: 992 Cal
- Fat: 101.65 g
- Protein: 2.9 g
- Sugar: 17.64 g

Oatmeal Raisin Cookies

Preparation Time: 10 minutes
Cooking Time: 25 minutes
Servings: 4

Ingredients:

✓ 1 cup of coconut oil
✓ 1 cup of coconut sugar or raw honey
✓ 1½ cups almond flour
✓ 1 tsp salt
✓ ½ tsp grated nutmeg
✓ 1 tsp cinnamon
✓ 1½ cups raisins
✓ 2 large eggs, well beaten
✓ 1 tbsp ground vanilla bean
✓ 3 cups rolled oats
✓ ½ cup chopped walnuts

Directions:

1. Heat oven to 350F.
2. Grease cookie sheets with coconut oil or line with waxed or parchment paper.
3. Mix coconut oil, coconut sugar or raw honey in a large bowl and beat until fluffy.
4. Add vanilla.
5. Beat in eggs.
6. Mix almond flour, salt, cinnamon, and nutmeg in a separate bowl.
7. Stir these dry ingredients into a fluffy mixture.
8. Mix in raisins and nuts.
9. Mix in oats.
10. Spoon out on cookie sheets, leaving 2-inches between cookies.
11. Bake until edges turn golden brown.

Nutrition:

✓ Calories: 400 Cal
✓ Fat: 27 g
✓ Protein: 61.86 g
✓ Sugar: 28 g

Coconut Cream Tart

Preparation Time: 10 minutes
Cooking Time: 30 minutes
Servings: 4

Ingredients:

Crust:

- ✓ 2 cups almonds, soaked overnight and drained
- ✓ 1 cup pitted dates, soaked overnight and drained
- ✓ 1 cup chopped dried apricots
- ✓ 1½ tsp ground vanilla bean
- ✓ 1 banana

Filling:

- ✓ 1 cup of flaked coconut
- ✓ 1 can of unsweetened coconut milk
- ✓ ¾ cup of raw honey
- ✓ 3 egg yolks
- ✓ 2 tbsp of arrowroot powder
- ✓ 2 tbsp of coconut oil
- ✓ 2 tsp of ground vanilla bean
- ✓ 1/8 tsp of salt
- ✓ ½ cup of coconut cream

Directions:

1. Heat the coconut milk, honey, salt and ground vanilla bean over medium heat in a medium-size saucepan.
2. In a separate bowl, whisk the egg yolks and arrowroot powder.
3. Add ½ cup of the warm coconut milk mixture to the egg yolks while whisking constantly. Then pour the egg mixture back into the coconut milk mixture and whisk until the mix thickens and then mix for 3 more minutes.
4. Take off of the heat and mix in the coconut oil and flaked coconut.
5. Cool and pour in the tart crust and refrigerate.
6. Decorate with large coconut flakes.

Nutrition:

- ✓ Calories: 325 Cal
- ✓ Fat: 23 g
- ✓ Protein: 35.76 g
- ✓ Sugar: 38 g

Apple Pie

Preparation Time: 10 minutes
Cooking Time: 35 minutes
Servings: 4

Ingredients:

For the crust:
- ✓ 2 Cups of almonds, drenched and drained overnight
- ✓ 1 Cup of pitted dates, soaked and drained overnight
- ✓ 1 Cup of dried apricots peeled
- ✓ 1 1⁄2 tsp of vanilla ground bean
- ✓ 1 Bananas 1

For Filling the Apple:
- ✓ 2 Tbsp olive oil
- ✓ 9 Apples sour, peeled, cored and cut into 1⁄4 "thick slices
- ✓ ¼ cup of coconut sugar or raw honey
- ✓ ½ tsp cinnamon
- ✓ 1/8 tsp sea salt
- ✓ ½ cup of coconut milk

For the topping:
- ✓ 1 cup ground nuts and seeds

Directions:
1. *Filling*: melt coconut oil in a large pot over medium heat.
2. Add apples, coconut sugar or raw honey, cinnamon and sea salt.
3. Increase heat to medium-high, and cook, stirring occasionally, until apples release their moisture and melted sugar.
4. Pour coconut milk or cream over apples and continue to cook until apples are soft and liquid has thickened, about 5 minutes, stirring occasionally.
5. Pour the filling into the crust and then top with topping.
6. To avoid burning place a pie shield over the edges of the crust.
7. Bake until topping is just turning golden brown.
8. Cool and serve.

Nutrition:
- ✓ Calories: 212 Cal
- ✓ Fat: 95.12 g
- ✓ Protein: 38.39 g
- ✓ Sugar: 26 g

Blueberry Cream Pie

Preparation Time: 10 minutes
Cooking Time: 30 minutes
Servings: 4

Ingredients:

- √ Sweet superfoods pie crust filling:
- √ 2 tsp plant-based gelatin, dissolved in 2 tbsp hot water
- √ 1/3 cup lemon juice
- √ 1/3 cup raw honey
- √ 1 can coconut milk, chilled
- √ 4 cups blueberries for serving

Directions:

1. Blend the gelatin and the water.
2. Add the lemon juice and stir to dissolve.
3. Whip some 15 minutes of coconut milk and raw honey with the electric mixer.
4. Stir in the whipped cream with the gelatin.
5. Pour the filling into the saucepan.
6. The filling is set in the fridge.
7. Chill until set at 4 hours, and serve with plenty of berries.

Nutrition:

- ✓ Calories: 210 Cal
- ✓ Fat: 52.62 g
- ✓ Protein: 19.61 g
- ✓ Sugar: 31 g

Mocha Chocolate Mousse

Everybody appreciates chocolate mousse and this one has a brilliant light and breezy surface. It is brisk and simple to make and is best served the day after it's made.

Preparation Time: 35 minutes
Cooking Time: 2 hours
Servings: 4-6

Ingredients:

- √   250g dim chocolate (85% cocoa solids)
- √   6 medium unfenced eggs, isolated
- √   4 tbsp solid dark espresso
- √   4 tbsp almond milk
- √   Chocolate espresso beans, to enrich

Directions:

1. Soften the chocolate in a huge bowl set over a skillet of delicately stewing water, ensuring the base of the bowl doesn't contact the water. Expel the bowl from the heat and leave the dissolved chocolate to cool to room temperature.
2. When the softened chocolate is at room temperature, race in the egg yolks each in turn and afterwards tenderly overlap in the espresso and almond milk.
3. Utilizing a hand-held electric blender, whisk the egg whites until firm pinnacles structure, at that point blend several tablespoons into the chocolate blend to release it. Delicately overlap in the rest of, an enormous metal spoon.
4. Move the mousse to singular glasses and smooth the surface. Spread with stick film and chill for in any event 2 hours, preferably medium-term. Enliven with chocolate espresso beans before serving.

Nutrition:

- ✓ Calories: 112 Cal
- ✓ Fat: 29.89 g
- ✓ Protein: 40.3 g
- ✓ Sugar: 128.13 g

Mediterranean Scones

Preparation Time: 10 minutes
Cooking Time: 10 minutes
Servings: 4

Ingredients:
For the scones:
- ✓ 250 g of flour
- ✓ 1 teaspoon of baking soda
- ✓ 2 teaspoons of cream of tartar
- ✓ 40 g of butter
- ✓ 150 ml of milk
- ✓ 1 egg
- ✓ salt
- ✓ black pepper

For the stuffing:
- ✓ 2 mozzarella cheese
- ✓ 1 red pepper
- ✓ 4 spoons of olives
- ✓ 3 spoons of desalted capers
- ✓ basil
- ✓ flax seed
- ✓ oil
- ✓ salt

Directions:
1. We prepare the scones by mixing the baking soda and cream of tartar with the flour. We combine a pinch of salt, plenty of black pepper, the cold butter into chunks and knead quickly to obtain a sandy mixture. We add the lightly beaten egg and mix, then we also add the milk, all at once. We mix the mixture and put it on a floured surface. We form 10 little balls bigger than a walnut and we crush them arranging them on a baking sheet. Bake at 220 ° C for about 10 minutes.
2. We cut the peppers into strips and sauté them in the pan with the oil and basil, add salt. We toast the flax seeds in a pan. We divide the scones in half and we will make them with mozzarella, peppers, olives and capers. Add a drizzle of oil and a sprinkling of flax seeds and cook again in the oven for a few minutes before serving.

Nutrition: Calories: 137 Cal | Fat: 48.32 g | Protein: 36.35 g | Sugar: 4.16 g

Chapter 20: Exercises to Do

The Sirtfood Diet is designed to help you activate your sirtuin genes without the necessity of exercise or fasting, but that doesn't mean you shouldn't add regular and consistent physical activity to your life to protect your body from deterioration and aging in other ways.

Your nutrition can do the lion's share of maintaining health and preventing disease but if you don't use your body and muscles on a regular basis, they will atrophy, stiffen up and stop working for you.

What this means primarily is that exercise doesn't have to be your go-to solution for weight loss or weight management, but rather it should be practiced as a means of maintaining our ability to move and stay strong and energetic. Our bodies were designed to go through a wide range of movements, from the bending, pulling and lifting required to farm, gather and harvest, to the cardiovascular capacity to hunt and the combination of all of the above that is required to keep children occupied and safe.

In short, even if a Sirtfood Diet helps you fight disease and reach your ideal body weight, you shouldn't neglect your exercise.

Moderate Movement

Walking is one type of physical activity that is considered moderate and most people are able to do it, though distance and speed may vary.

You've probably heard of the social movement in which people around the world are encouraged to track their steps and work towards a goal of 10,000 steps a day.

One study looked at a healthy, youthful population of students and asked one group to meet these 10,000 steps per day goal and another group to simplify their lives with elevators, wheelchairs, and plenty of sitting, reducing their steps per day to a mere 2,000 steps. Within 2 weeks, the less active group lost an average of 5% of their muscle mass (TEDx, 2014).

As a society, many of us are not even reaching 2,000 steps per day.
You're reading this because you want to change your life through your diet, and sirtfoods are beautifully designed to help you do just that. It would be a mistake, however, to think that you don't still have to spend some of your time each day moving your body.

The reality is that humans were designed to eat nutritiously in order to move effectively. If we eliminate either or both of those factors from the equation of our lives, we are going to feel the effects in the form of disease, weight gain and the breakdown of our bodies. Being able to move is a joy that we should not take for granted.

With the Sirtfood Diet in your corner, there should be no need to exercise as a means of keeping your weight at an optimal level, however, it can help you find that level more quickly.

From the start, this has been more about creating and maintaining health for you, rather than simply focusing on weight. If we look at all the chronic diseases that we're trying to prevent, such as heart disease, diabetes, and cancer, we should be doing anything we can think of to prevent these tragic conditions from claiming our lives.

There's almost unlimited scientific evidence that physical activity can reduce your risk for all of these diseases. We know that a large part of that protection is because our sirtuin genes are activated. Just because sirtfoods can also activate those genes doesn't mean we should assume physical activity is no longer necessary.

Instead, we should consider the compounded benefits of integrating both a sirtfood rich diet with moderate physical activity on a regular basis.

We should be enjoying the gift of movement more than anything, whenever we have the opportunity. It doesn't need to be an exhausting activity and you shouldn't hate doing it. It is supposed to make you feel energized, relaxed and content. Government guidelines suggest a mere 2.5 hours of moderate activity per week that works out to less than 30 minutes per day. Moderate activity can be almost anything you enjoy doing, walking your dog or joining an adult amateur sports team.

You will want to monitor your physical activity to some extent during the first phase of the Sirtfood Diet, because you will consume less calories than your body is used to No need to put your body under more stress. But as described here moderate movement can absolutely enhance your first-stage experience and results.

Once you're consuming a regular number of calories again, but enjoying the significantly improved health benefits of a diet loaded with sirtfoods, you're even encouraged to increase your current physical activity to add more long-term health to your life.

Muscle and Strength

When you're completely sedentary, doing nothing but lounging in front of your television or working at a computer desk, your muscles require about 30% of the energy your body needs to keep you just sitting there.

When you exercise, your muscles use closer to 90% of your energy. As you can imagine, this will burn up a lot more carbohydrates and fat than simply sitting in your chair, but you knew that already.

The less you use your muscles, the smaller and weaker they will get but again, this is not news.

Why is muscle mass and strength so important to our health?

One reason is that studies show that the risk of death for individuals classified as "strong" is about half that of those classified as "weak" amongst all causes of mortality. The stronger you are, the more likely you are to remain alive. That is definitely motivating.

65 It's not old and we should all expect to live that long at least, and many of us are much longer.

But 65 years of inactivity is a long time to let your muscles shrink, and this is a major contributing factor to chronic disease prevalence at this age.

One particular shocking disease is sarcopenia, which is the age-related waste of our muscles. As we age, after reaching our 30s, we naturally start losing muscle mass and strength at a rate of about 3 percent or more per decade. This is, besides the muscle, that we simply lose from being sedentary. Usually, that muscles traded in for fat.

Muscle mass is not purely designed for aesthetic purposes. It is associated with both our balance and our bone density, which can lead to frailty and loss of independence in our future.

But it isn't just in our retirement years that a lack of muscle will start to really affect us. Diseases such as cancer, renal failure, heart disease, and rheumatoid and osteoarthritis are all linked to lower muscle mass, both as a cause and as a result.

We know sirtfoods can help protect our muscle mass, but how should we build it?
The moderate movement suggestions are ideal during the first phase of the Sirtfood Diet, or any time in your life you 're reducing calories for any other reason. But we will need to dedicate more energy specifically to our muscles to live a full, healthy, and strong life.

Our bodies are designed to adapt to what transforms into a normal motion. If you've never gone into your life before for a jog, the first block will be a fight. But if you practice every day, your body will adapt and it will become easy to jog 1 block.

If you have never lifted a baby before and you find yourself having to carry one around for 8 -10 hours a day, even a tiny 7-pound newborn is going to feel heavy at first. But after a few weeks of parenthood, your body will adapt, you will become stronger, and even when your baby weighs 20 pounds, you won't find them too heavy to manage.

We are not all going to be carrying around growing babies all our lives, however, so a smart way to grow your muscles using the same principle is to either lift weights or use your bodyweight.

Using weights gives you the ability to track any improvements in strength as you find yourself progressively adding more weight to your lifting. However, bodyweight exercises have the distinct advantage of not requiring any equipment and they use dynamic movements, which also help to improve total body wellness, flexibility, and mobility.

Bodyweight exercises include movements like pushups, pullups, squats, and lunges, taking the stairs and even holding much yoga poses.

You don't have to give your entire life over to becoming an athlete. You can see dramatic results in as little as 3 days a week, only 30 minutes at a time.

If you begin progressively building strength from a younger age, you will protect yourself against many so-called chronic and age-related diseases. If you are already in the range of 65+ years of age, all is not lost.

If you start challenging your muscles now, with your doctor's permission and guidance, you can build them up again and start recovering from any muscle loss-related illnesses you may already have. You will need to start slowly and carefully, but in just a few weeks of training, the results can quickly change your outlook on life.

A Sirtfood diet will help to protect the muscle you have, but to really combat this natural process, you should be dedicated to actively strengthening your muscles throughout your entire life. Lifting weights or doing progressively more challenging bodyweight exercises is a great way to build your muscles.

Chapter 21: Phase One Meal Plan

Phase 1: 7 pounds in 7 days

The phase 1 of the Sirtfood diet is the one that will allow you to take the first successful step towards achieving a leaner shape and a healthier glow.

The authors of the diet proved with their clinical trial, that no matter your initial weight or gender, you will lose 7 pounds in 7 days, and it won't be muscle mass!
This is actually not the most amazing part of the diet, the fact that the lost pounds won't come back to haunt you is! After all, the first week of the diet is based on the simple, well-proven base of calorie restriction, but with the added twist of a sirtfood-laden meal plan.

Not only will you see an improvement of your shape, but you will feel more vital, your skin will achieve a natural glow that no cream can ever compete with. I was skeptical at first too, but I never felt so energetic, clean, and beautiful.

Phase 1 of the diet is the one that produces the greatest results. Over the course of seven days, you will follow a simple method in order to lose 3.5 kg.
During the first three days, the intake of calories will have to be limited to one thousand per day at most. Basically, you can have three green juices and a solid meal, all based on Sirt foods. From day 4 to 7, the daily calories will become fifteen hundred. Every day you will eat two green juices and two solid Sirt-meals.

By the end of the seven days, you should have lost, on average, 3.5 kilos.
Despite the reduction in calories, the participants do not feel hungry, and the calorie limit is an indication rather than a goal. Even in the most intensive phase, calorie restriction is not as drastic as in many other regimes. Sirtfoods have a naturally satiating effect so that many of you will feel pleasantly full and satisfied.

Phase 1 plan:

Days 1 to 3 – max. 1000 calories

- ✓ 3 green juices
- ✓ 1 main Sirtfood meal

Think of this first 3 days as the reset button for your metabolism. I swear it isn't as grueling as it seems. The match in the green juice and the SIRT-activating of the foods will satisfy and make you feel more energetic than ever.

Days 4 to 7 – max. 1500 calories

- ✓ 2 Green juices
- ✓ 2 main Sirtfood meals

Tips to get started

1. Get a good juicer

One necessary kitchen tool that you will need aside from the actual foods is a juicer. You will need a juicer as soon as you start the Sirtfood diet. Juicers are everywhere so they are quite easy to find, but the quality ranges greatly, however.

This is where price, function, and convenience come into play. You could go to a popular department store, or you can find them online. Once you know what you are going after, you can shop around.

The quality of the juicer will also determine the nutritional quality and sometimes the taste of your juice, which we will explain in a bit. Just know that buying a cheap juicer may seem like a good idea now, but if you decide to upgrade then you will have spent more money, and twice. If you buy a good juicer, think of it as an investment into your health. Many people have spent money on a gym membership that went unused for quadruple the cost of one juicer. A juicer won't go to waste.

Note: If all else fails, in a pinch and with a blender you could get away with an (albeit very poor quality) juice by blending the foods, and using a fine mesh to filter the juice that is left. The only problem is that you would be getting a fraction of the nutrients, and also probably a spike in sugar, as very little fiber will be in the juice to help slow down the natural sugar absorption. Use caution.

2. Stock your fridge and pantry

First, clear your cabinets and refrigerator of foods that are obviously unhealthy and that might tempt you. You also will have a very low-calorie intake at the start, and you do not want to be tempted into a quick fix that may set you back. Even though you will have new recipes, you may feel that your old comfort foods are easier at the moment.

Then, go shopping for all of the ingredients that you will need for the week. If you buy what you will need it is more cost-effective. Also, once you see the recipes, you will notice that there are many ingredients that overlap. You will get to know your portions as you proceed with the diet but at least you will have what you need and save yourself some trips to the store.

Wash, dry, cut and store all of the foods that you need, that way you have them conveniently prepared when you need them. This will make a new diet seem less tedious.

3.   Prepare in advance

A resolution for a change in diet is often thwarted by the lack of time. So, knowing this, prepare. You can easily prepare the meals the night before to take to work the day after instead of getting tempted by a cafeteria sandwich. Juices can be prepared in bulk and stored. They will keep in the fridge for 3 days and even longer in the freezer. It is very important that you protect them from light and add the matcha only when you are ready to consume them.

4.   Get used to eating early

Drink your juices as the earlier meals in the day if it helps you. For three reasons: It's a great way to start your day. (1) It will give you energy for breakfast and for lunch especially. By not having to digest heavy foods, your body saves time and energy usually spent on moving things around to go through all the laborious motions. You will be guaranteed to feel lighter and more energetic this way. You can always change this pattern after the maintenance phase, but you may find that you want to keep that schedule. (2) Having fruits and vegetables before starchy or cooked meals, no matter how healthy the ingredients, is the best way to go for your digestion. Fruits and vegetables digest more rapidly, and the breakdown into the compounds that we can use more readily. Think of it as having your salad before your dinner. It works in the same way. The heavier foods, grains, oils, meats, etc., take more time to digest. If you eat these first, they will slow things down and that is where you have a backup of food needing to be broken down. This is also when you may find yourself with indigestion. (3)

Juices, especially green juices contain phytochemicals that not only serve as anti-oxidants but they contribute to our energy and mood. You will notice that you feel much differently after drinking a green juice than you would if you had eggs and sausage. You may want to make a food diary and note things such as this!

Even without following the Sirtfood diet, eating early in the day is the healthier choice. Our busy lives often don't allow for a proper breakfast, but Sirtfoods give some great option for a quick breakfast on-the-go (smoothies, pre-prepared muesli, easy scrambled eggs and tofu). Sirtfoods supercharge our energies, so you have all the more to gain by getting them early in the morning. The day won't feel quite as long as it used to!

5.   Be mindful of what you are drinking

Besides the mandatory green juices, you should feel free to drink freely: plain water, black coffee, and green tea are recommended. Do not drink soft drinks and fruit juices! To make your water tastier and more "SIRT-full" you can add some sliced strawberries to cold sparkling water.

Don't change your coffee habits: caffeine withdrawal can be grueling and, likewise, you shouldn't start drinking it if you are not a habitual consumer. Do try to drink your coffee black. Clinical researchers have discovered that milk can impair the absorption of the SIRT-activating nutrients, the same goes for green tea. Add a slice of lemon to your green tea instead it will increase the absorption of the nutrients that stimulate SIRT.

For this first week include red wine only as a cooking ingredient.

6.   Eat until you are 80% full

It's an Okinawan proverb and it couldn't be truer. Sirtfoods will more than satisfy your appetite, you might even find yourself feeling full before finishing your meal, don't force it down!

7.   Think of the journey and not the destination

This is not a diet to lose weight, it's a change in lifestyle and a celebration of the most diverse culinary traditions. Take joy in cooking and knowing that you are eating well. Focus on the path, rather than the destination and you will find it much easier to follow the diet.

Phase Two Meal Plan

This part of the first week is less radical than the other one, but it involves lowering your green juice intake from three servings to just two. You can have one green juice at 9:00 a.m., and the second one at 4:00 p.m. (for instance), but you can adjust the schedule according to your time.
But don't worry. As you will compensate with an extra main meal, you will have two meals per day during this phase. You should be able to keep the same dessert (the dark chocolate with 85 percent cocoa), and you will have again the option to choose from a standard or vegan meal.

Day 4

For this day, you will have included in your menu two standard meals and two vegan meals. You can choose to have both meals standard or both meals vegan, but if you want to mix them (to have one meal vegan and the other one standard), feel free to do so. You can have your breakfast at 7:00 a.m. and the second meal at 1:00 p.m.

Therefore, these are the standard meals: sirt muesli, which is a proper breakfast meal, and salmon fillet with caramelized endive, celery leaf, and arugula salad. (Don't forget to pour some extra-virgin olive oil on the salad.)

As for the vegan meals, you can have sirt muesli (vegan style) and Tuscan bean stew.

Day 5

For this day, you can stick to the same juice drinking and eating schedule. The only difference is that you are trying different meals than the day before.
For the standard diet, you can have strawberry buckwheat tabbouleh and stir-fried greens with miso-marinated baked cod. For the vegan menu, you can try vegan strawberry buckwheat tabbouleh and buckwheat noodles in miso broth with celery, kale, and tofu.

Day 6

There isn't too much difference between day 6 and the prior days of phase 2. Just stick to the same green juices and the same schedule for having them, or you can have the meals.

When it comes to the standard food preference, you can have sirt super salad and grilled beef with herb-roasted potatoes, onion rings, garlic kale, and red wine. (Now this sounds too delicious, so you have to try it.)

But if you are not into beef, then perhaps you want to go with the vegan menu: lentil sirt super salad and baked potato with kidney bean mole.

Day 7

You are finishing the seven-day meal plan in style, as this day has included extremely delicious meals. You already have the scheduled set for your meals and green juices, plus you still have a small piece of dark chocolate (after each meal) to sweeten your day (not that it requires sweetening).

If you want to choose the standard meals, you can go with the sirtfood omelet, baked chicken breast with walnut, and red onion and parsley pesto salad (some extra-virgin olive oil is recommended). If you feel like you want to try the vegan menu, you can have vegan Waldorf salad and roasted eggplant wedges with walnut and tomato and parsley pesto salad (don't forget to add extra-virgin olive oil).

The menu suggested during these days can be used as guidelines, but it is up to you if you want to stick to having these meals exactly on the same days as mentioned in the plan. Perhaps you want to try the meal from day 1 on day 3, and the other way around. I wouldn't recommend trying a meal from day 5 or day 6 in phase 1 of the seven-day meal plan. Therefore, feel free to play with the meals, but make sure you don't have a meal that is for phase 2 of the first week in phase 1 or the other way around. You will need to pay attention to quantity as well.

These foods may sound delicious, but you can't have a huge portion. You really need to stick with the quantity mentioned in the recipes. Speaking of recipes, I mentioned some standard and vegan meals, but I haven't said anything about how to prepare them. Well, don't worry! This collection will have plenty of recipes you can use during this meal plan.

Conclusion

When you first switch to a clean diet it can be difficult to understand which foods are clean foods and which ones are not. When buying fresh foods always aim for the organic varieties, but if this is not possible then any fresh food is better than the processed option.

To help you plan your food shopping, the following lists show a variety of clean foods which you can incorporate into your meal plans.

Fresh Fruit & Vegetables
➢ All varieties of fresh fruit and vegetables, including raw, frozen fruit and vegetables should be incorporated into your clean diet to ensure a good variety of natural vitamins and minerals. If possible, buy organic produce as it is free from pesticides.
➢ Although most fruits contain sugar, this is a natural sugar and far healthier than the refined sugars found in processed foods.

Meat & Fish
All types of meat and fish are suitable for a clean diet but there are a few guidelines you should be aware of.
➢ **Beef:** This is best to buy directly from a butcher as you should choose only grass-fed and humanely raised beef.
➢ **Pork:** The majority of pork products are processed so avoid ham and cheaper cuts of pork, gammon and bacon. Stick to only the high-quality pork options. Again, a butcher's is the best place to purchase pork as you can gain information as to its quality.
➢ **Fish:** Always buy fish that has been caught sustainably and limit high mercury content fish to 2 servings per week.

High mercury content fish includes:
- *King Mackerel*
- *Marlin*
- *Shark*
- *Swordfish*
- *Tuna*

Poultry & Eggs
All eggs and poultry are a good source of protein but choose the free-range, organic options whenever possible.

Many of the cheaper super store varieties of fresh chicken will have added water which cannot be considered as clean food.
Check for products that state no added water or even salt!

Dairy Products

> **Milk:** Always choose full-fat varieties and stick to organic milk whenever possible. For a clean alternative, you could switch to pure, unsweetened, organic coconut milk, canned varieties not cartons, or unsweetened organic soy milk.

> **Cheese:** Block cheeses only and full-fat varieties. Never buy pre-shredded cheeses or low-fat version and stick to the better-quality cheeses.

> **Cottage Cheese:** Only good quality, full-fat varieties.

> **Yoghurt:** Full-fat plain yoghurts. If you prefer flavored yoghurt mix a little whole or pureed fruit into the plain yoghurt.

Beans, Pulses & Seeds

All beans, lentils, chickpeas etc. can be included in recipes
For a little variety to your recipes try adding sunflower, flax or sesame seeds.

Unrefined Grains

> **Wheat:** Use whole meal varieties of bread, pasta and rice. If possible, stick to organic.

> **Oats:** Use unflavored rolled oats or steel-cut oats in recipes.

> **Flour:** Always use whole wheat flours when cooking and for an alternative to wheat you can use unprocessed coconut or almond flour.

Cooking Oils

Choose natural oils such as Olive Oil, Coconut oil, and Avocado Oil.

Herbs & Spices

Always choose fresh or dried herbs and spices and avoid seasoning packets. I would recommend spending a little time and money stocking a great herbs and spice store at home. They will come in so handy when preparing clean meals.

Natural Sweeteners

> **Honey:** Organic when possible
> **Pure syrup:** Avoid processed bottles and buy organic where possible.

Condiments

> ➤ Always choose no added sugar varieties

> ➤ **Ketchup & Mustard:** It is possible to purchase clean varieties but these are often very difficult to find. The cleanest option is to make your own.

Thank you for reading!

I hope that you find the success you are looking for.

I hope this guide has helped you become acquainted with the Sirtfood diet and achieve your weight loss and health goals.

Good luck on your sirtfood journey!

|BOOK 2|

Mediterranean Diet Cookbook For Beginners 2021

70+ Fresh and Foolproof Recipes with 21-Day Meal Plan for a Healthy Lifestyle

Introduction

If you have ever noticed the health of people today, especially teenagers, and the food items that fill their platter, you may not take much time to find the type of health they possess. Their little, partial or full obesity may find its reason in pizza, white bread, refined sugar, processed food they eat which has many preservatives. The taste buds seem to reign supreme in the kingdom of food.

But the analysis and research on processed food items like frozen food, white bread and carbonated drinks, has brought startling facts forward. It has surfaced in some of the research findings that huge and habitual consumption of these items can tax the body. Its over consumption can result in high production of insulin. This can cause the risk of diabetes, obesity and coronary malfunction.

The reality of animal fat is not much different. The saturated fats in these food items can have adverse effect on our body. It causes accumulation of extra fats in our body and disturbs our body mass index. The saturated fat in animal products milk and butter increases bad cholesterol-LDL. In short, it can harm coronary health

In this technologically advanced when with little efforts we can accomplish our tasks. Physical activities are negligible. Poor health comfortably steps in. It becomes essential to switch to healthier diet which fulfils the nutrition need of our body and at the same time keeps us filled. There is much information on nutrition filled diet. However, it is difficult to make a choice.

Nonetheless when we have visible effects of centuries, over generations of people, we can trust it to some extent. A nutrition analysis can help make our trust stay longer in it. This is true about Mediterranean diet. A food pattern which brims with whole grains, plant based diet has olive oil as a source of fats and other items which provide calories essential for our body. This diet has no space for processed food is loaded with sugar or artificial sweeteners. As a result the low amount of fats keeps the heart healthy, provides both the essential nutrients and agility. Give it a start, I feel you won't look back. You will rather leap into a healthy future.

"Wish you a healthy eating."

What is Mediterranean Diet?

When one reads the word Mediterranean, one tends to think nothing but of sea. Thinking of a vast sea brings to mind the sea food. When its history is looked into, it transpires that it has its roots in Mediterranean basin, a land which has been historically called a powerhouse of societal evolution of the world. As here the social history of whole world may be lying stored. This area in Nile valley was a good land for the people of East and West. The frequent interaction of people from different regions and culture had larger effect on customs, languages, religion, perspective, and had transformative effect on life style. This cultural integration and clash further had an effect on eating habit too.

Looking at the food content of Mediterranean diet one can see the reflection of diverse culture and class. Bread, wine and oil reflect village and agriculture; this is further complemented by vegetable like lettuce, mushroom, mallow and little preference for meat but much preference for fish and sea food. This shows the gluttonous nature of people from Rome. Here we also get Germanic flavour of pig's meat with garden vegetables. The beer was made with grains.

The food culture of bread, wine and oil went beyond Germanic and Christian Roman culture and entered the boundaries of Arabs. The reason was their existence at the southern shore of the Mediterranean. Their food culture was unique because of the variety of leafy vegetables they grew. They had egg plants, spinach, sugarcane, and fruits like oranges, citrus, lemon, and pomegranate and resembled rose water of the European cuisine. This had an influence on the cooking style of Latin and affect the recipes.

The big geographical event that is discovery of America by European has great additional impact on Mediterranean diet. This event added a range of new foodstuffs like beans, potatoes, tomatoes, chilli and peppers. Tomato, the red plant, was first ornamental and later was considered edible. It further became an important part of Mediterranean diet.

The historical analysis of Mediterranean diet shows how from feeding of Egyptian to discovery of America gave us the Mediterranean diet of the today. The nutritional model of Mediterranean diet is kept so much in high commendation that it is related to cultural, social, and environmental that it is intimately related to Mediterranean people, their lifestyle and history.

There are some established health and cultural platforms like UNESCO which define Mediterranean diet unfolding the meaning of word diet which has come from the word 'diata' that means lifestyle, a way of life. It focuses on the journey of food from landscape to the table; covering cuisine, harvesting, processing, preparation, fishing, cooking and a specific way of consumption.

There is a variation in Mediterranean diet in different countries due to ethnic and cultural differences, diverse religion and economic disparity. As per the description and recommendation of dietician and food experts the Mediterranean diet has the following proportion of foods. In cereals there are whole grains and legumes. For fats olive oil is a major source. Onion, garlic, tomatoes and leafy vegetables and peppers are major greens. Fresh fruits are major in snacks and desserts. Eggs, milk, yogurt and other dairy products are taken moderately. The food items like red meat, processed food, refined sugar are taken as little as possible.

This diet has 25 % to 35% proportion of fat content of the calorie count and saturated fat is never beyond 8 %. As far as oil is concerned there are region-wise alternatives. In central and northern Italy butter and lard are commonly used in cooking. Olive is mainly used for snacks and salad dressing.

This diet reflect food pattern of Crete, rest of Greece and much part of Italy in early 1960. It gained widespread recognition in 1990s. There is an irony in Mediterranean diet although people living in this region have a tendency to consume high amount of fats but they enjoy far better cardiovascular health as compared to people of America who consume equal amount of fat.

The tradition of Mediterranean diet offers cuisine rich in colour, taste, flavour and aroma. Most of all it keeps us closer to nature. It may be simple in looks but rich in health and has much to offer that is no way less than any other healthy diet. Some Americans describe Mediterranean diet as all styles of homemade pasta with Parmesan sauce and enrichment with a few pieces of meat is pretty occasional. That too for replacing beans and macaroni. It has omnipresence of so many fresh vegetables with just olive oil sprinkled. And desserts in this diet have nothing but always fresh fruits.

However, a good Mediterranean diet does not include ever soybean oil, canola or any other refined oil. There is no room for processed meat, refined sugar, white bread, refined grains or white pasta or pizza dough containing white flour.

This diet is characterised with a balanced use of food items which have high amount of fibre, unsaturated fats and antioxidants. Besides, there is an approach which gives health a priority by cutting the consumption of unhealthy animal fats and meat. This strikes a balance between the amount of energy intake and its consumption.

This magical diet is not just a preferential health food, with a wide range of magical recipes but also a conduit between wide ranges of cultures. People of this region are son of the soil and so is their food that comes from land and soil. It can ensure, if consumed rationally, efficacy of different bodily functions.

Some famous health organisations across the globe have designed food pyramids to make it clear what are the most common forms of Mediterranean region. It became popular among health activists because people of this region have high life expectancy despite less access to health facilities. It has been recommended by American Heart Association and American Diabetes Association that Mediterranean diet lowers the risk of cardiovascular disease and type two diabetes. If a patterned Mediterranean diet plan is followed, it may have a lasting effect on health and can help in reducing and maintaining healthy weight.

What are the benefits of Mediterranean Diet?

In this nutrition and health conscious world medical scientists, nutritionists and health scientists keep researching for healthy options and lifestyle changes which can ensure health and longevity along with agility. There is an emerging consensus among health experts that a diet which has fibre, balanced amount of protein, healthy fats and minerals can lead to optimum health and a healthy life.

It can check cardiovascular diseases, diabetes, cancer, stroke and help in maintaining healthy weight. Mediterranean diet has all these attributes. Its ingredients are rich in plants, healthy fats, fruits, whole grains, healthy meat and much more. As a matter of fact, it has all the elements which are essential to a healthy diet. There has been claims about its positive effect on health and physical well-being.

In a study conducted over 25000 women across a period of 12 years it has been established that those who consume Mediterranean diet has 25 percent less chances of having any cardiovascular

disease. The reason behind this positive change is decline in inflammation, glucose level in blood and an improved body mass index.

There is low saturated fat with high amount of monosaturated fats, protein and dietary fibre. Its olive oil has a major healthy element that is oleic acid. It is highly beneficial for the health of human heart. **It has the approval of European Food Safety Authority** Panel on Dietetic Products, Nutrition and Allergies. It has been mentioned that its polyphenols protects the oxidation of lipids in blood. It happens because of priority being given to olive oil which has oleic acid that helps in maintaining normal LDL level in blood and may check cardiovascular diseases. This has been claimed by American Heart Association as well that consumption of olive oil can be an aid to maintaining cardiovascular health. If this diet is followed the intake of refined breads, processed foods and unhealthy meat gets reduced, on the other hand it recommends replacing hard liquor with red wine. This way it can reduce the risk of cardiovascular diseases.

This diet has high fiber content. This reduces glucose level in blood and checks the causes which develop type 2 diabetes. This fiber makes one feel full and keep eating cravings under control.

This also helps in keeping weight under check and reduces constipation and helps regulate bowel movement.

Maintaining healthy weight is key factor to good health. It becomes easy to maintain an ideal weight when a fruit and vegetable rich diet is taken. The icing on the cake is total absence of refined sugar and white floor. A physical routine if is combined with it, it becomes easy to maintain a healthy weight. This may help in reducing obesity as well. Moreover, maintaining an ideal weight can give us multiple health benefits.

It has been found through a comprehensive research that a regular and monitored consumption of Mediterranean diet can reduce the risk of death from cancer by five to six percent. This has been confirmed in a study conducted on cancer patients in 2017. It has also been found that it may decrease the chances of cancer.

Stress is the key factor of affecting life adversely today. Mediterranean diet can be a relaxant here. It has been found in various studies that a sincere adherence to Mediterranean diet can check the impairment of cognitive ability. It does so by improving good cholesterol, levels of blood sugar and overall health of blood vessels. This as a result reduce your risk of dementia or Alzheimer's disease.

Mediterranean diet with maximum vegetables, fruits and nuts in it, is rich with antioxidants, vitamins and other nutrients. This helps cells form going through any damaging process. This damage otherwise occurs if there is an oxidative stress. Consequently, it reduces the risk of Parkinson's disease by fifty percent. Adhering to this diet can also lower the causes of depression and give a healthier state of mind.

It has been noticed in a study conducted by food scientists over women who had chances of stroke in United Kingdom. When they followed Mediterranean diet very strictly it reduced their chances of getting stroke by twenty percent. However, it was not so in men. But the clinical researches are underway to observe its effect on the male gender as well.

National Institute on Aging funded a small study on aging which was published on 2018. In the journal it was highlighted, how looking at brain scan of 70 persons it was found that the people who strictly adhered to Mediterranean diet did not show any sign of aging. While those who had preference for other forms of diet had a plaque pattern which adds the adverse effect of aging. This shows that Mediterranean diet adds longevity to human life and gives lasting health.

Lungs play an important role in oxygenating our body but with age its inhalation ability impairs. The whole grains, dairy products and fish can improve the ability of lungs to perform better. Further, those who remain disciplined and steadfast in taking Mediterranean diet has 22-29 percent less chances of getting hearing loss.

It is an obvious fact that Mediterranean diet has an ample amount of nutrients and if we consume this diet it helps in prevention of muscle damage and boost the muscle strength and enhances agility. This improves efficiency of brain. This means consumers of this diet have better thinking and learning abilities, an improved memory and much better concentration.

This diet is quite beneficial for kidney patients and those who for some reason have to undergo kidney transplant. In studies, it has been found that it can reduce the risk of kidney dysfunction. Further, it can bring down graft failure by as much as thirty two percent and its loss by twenty six percent in the patients who undergo kidney transplant.

If a person develops inflammatory bowel diseases like piles, Mediterranean diet can cause a cure. It has been found after studies and preparing case histories that consumer of this diet are 57 percent less prone to develop Crohn's disease.

How to get started?

The best way to cause a change is to start it. But the biggest question that always awaits its answer is the way to start. Nonetheless the situation is much better if what we are to start has multiple benefits. Mediterranean diet obviously falls in this category where advantages outnumber the limitations, it may force on our lifestyle.
If you feel that it is difficult to change your diet, you can choose alternatives which really work well and can help switching to healthier option. Here are certain ways that can help switch to Mediterranean diet.

It is good to start by keeping vegetables and fruits at the upper ladder in your list of priorities and giving sausages and pepperoni in salad dressing a backseat. You can start by giving a plate of tomato slices a try. It should be just given a drizzle of olive oil and meshed feta cheese. Soups, crudité plates and salads can be awesome starters.
Skipping breakfast may seem effective but it can put extra burden on your system to keep you going. On the contrary, whole grains, fruits and other foods which are rich in fibre can be an effective way to start your day. Moreover, it will keep you filled and your cravings at a bay.

Replacing usual calorie loaded desserts like cake, ice cream, pastries etc. with fruits like apples, grapes, fresh figs or strawberries. This will make you digest better and stay lighter. A refreshing feeling will work as a motivation and keep you adherent to this magical diet.
If you leap to change it may never happen. There is a famous saying, 'A thousand miles journey starts with a single step.' This is quite applicable to shifting to Mediterranean diet. You can start with small steps like sauté with olive oil, eat more vegetables and fruits by enjoying, in starter, some salad. Replace your snacks with fruits. Similarly, other heavy dishes can be substituted with veggies.

Preferring skimmed milk or milk with 2 percent fats over full fat milk. This will be making you feel lighter and healthier. As a result it will work as a motivating factor for opting Mediterranean diet. The change felt in energy level and the nutrition experienced will work as a triggering factor and a driving force.

It is said if it is easy, it is achievable. The most accessible is to use whole grains in place of refined grains. Your choice should be whole wheat bread and not white bread that is made of refined flour. Similarly, brown rice or wild rice should replace white rice. Sometimes it is difficult choose authentic whole grains. It is easy now as a black and gold stamp has been developed by Oldways Whole Grain Council to select quality over paste.

Ancient grains or whole grains form an important part of Mediterranean diet. There is a huge variety of these grains. These are amaranth, faro, millet, spelt, and the believably Egyptian, Kamut; yet another is teff, it is similar to poppy seed in its size. You can try one seed at a time. Slowly and steady you can move to more options. In other words, you can switch to the other variety of seeds. As each seed has its own flavour and texture. The good news is these whole grains have become quite popular and are quite common. Consequently, these are now available in mainstream restaurants as well. It means you can try it and then make it a part of your diet.

If you make up your mind to go for it. You should take at least six servings a day. Half of it should be of whole grains. It may be worrisome to some because of carbs. But you can throw your tension to winds because it, for sure, will cause long term benefits. You should not overlook the fact that quick loss of weight may not be healthy. So whole grain in Mediterranean diet is the best option.

You may not be able to swap your current diet with Mediterranean at once. So, one meal based on vegetables, whole grains and beans. Spices and herbs can be peppered with spices to add a palatable punch.

If you are protein conscious and remain worried about it in your diet. Your dependence on meat can end by giving room to lentils in your diet. As these are the sources of high protein and have much fibre too. Beans have an edge, as these have ample antioxidants too. How motivating!

If it is in your easy reach, it can be your easy preference. Stocking your pantry with handy ingredients. These ingredients should be easy to use. Some of these can be popular protein sources like lentils, chickpeas and beans. Lentils have only twenty five minutes of cooking time without any need of overnight soaking. As for chickpeas and canned beans, you only need to rinse and then you can just put them into soups, burgers, salads, sandwiches and much more.

Giving up meat altogether may be a challenge but you can give it a start by taking meat in small proportion. Using small pieces of chicken or lean meat slices. You can stir fry your dish and avoid deep fry. It will keep it less oil soaked and more nourishing. It is a good news for fish eater as when they are on Mediterranean diet they can eat two servings of salmon, sardines and tuna these are essential to Mediterranean diet at least twice a week. There may be a risk of mercury but in the opinion of American nutritionists here benefits outrun the risk. The variety of fish mentioned here has comparatively less amount of mercury.

Dairy products are also a great protein source. Yogurt if it is Greek and a cheese cube is something which those on Mediterranean diet are encouraged to eat. But it should be in moderation.

In short, Mediterranean diet is a healthy option with wide range of tasty choices. If you start with an easy approach taking small steps at a time. Making little changes in your meal plans, you can go a long way.

21 Days Meal Plan

DAYS	Breakfast	Lunch	Snacks	Dinner
Day 1	Spinach and Artichoke Frittata	Mediterranean Chickpea Quinoa Bowl	15 Minute Mediterranean Chickpea Salad	Mediterranean Portobello Mushroom Pizzas with Arugula Salad
Day 2	Hearty Breakfast Fruit Salad	Harissa Chickpea Stew With Eggplant and Millet	Lemon Herb Mediterranean Pasta Salad	Slow-Cooker Mediterranean Quinoa with Arugula
Day 3	Shakshuka	Five-Minute Heirloom Tomato Toast	Hummus	Walnut-Rosemary Crusted Salmon
Day 4	Balsamic Berries with Honey Yogurt	Eggplant and Herb Flatbread	Mini Greek Pita Pizzas	Mediterranean Stuffed Chicken Breasts
Day 5	Caprese Avocado Toast	15-Minute Mediterranean Couscous with Tuna and Pepperoncini	Healthy Avocado Cilantro White Bean Dip	Charred Shrimp & Pesto Buddha Bowls
Day 6	Spinach Feta Breakfast Wraps	Pesto Quinoa Bowls With Roasted Veggies and Labneh	Homemade Granola Bars Recipe (Gluten-Free, Vegan, Dairy-Free)	Sheet-Pan Salmon with Sweet Potatoes & Broccoli

Day 7	Easy Homemade Muesli	Greek Yogurt Chicken Salad Stuffed Peppers	Peach Caprese Skewers	Greek Cauliflower Rice Bowls with Grilled Chicken
Day 8	Kale and Goat Cheese Frittata Cups	15-Minute Mezze Plate with Toasted Za'atar Pita Bread	Charcuterie Bistro Lunch Box	Prosciutto Pizza with Corn & Arugula
Day 9	Easy, Fluffy Lemon Ricotta Pancakes	Greek Lemon Chicken Skewers With Tzatziki Sauce	Hummus, Feta & Bell Pepper Cracker	Vegan Mediterranean Lentil Soup
Day 10	Smashed Egg Toasts with Herby Lemon Yogurt	Eggplant Pizza	Tomato-Basil Skewers	BBQ Shrimp with Garlicky Kale & Parmesan - Herb Couscous
Day 11	Mediterranean Breakfast Pitas	Cold Lemon Zooldes	Marinated Olives & Feta	Green Shakshuka with Spinach, Chard & Feta
Day 12	Crispy White Beans with Greens and Poached Egg	Stuffed Eggplant	Garlic Hummus	One-Skillet Salmon with Fennel & Sun-Dried Tomato Couscous
Day 13	Breakfast Grain Salad with Blueberries, Hazelnuts & Lemon	Wild Alaska Salmon and Smashed Cucumber Grain Bowls	Clementine & Pistachio Ricotta	Chicken & Spinach Skillet Pasta with Lemon & Parmesan
Day 14	Eggs with Summer Tomatoes, Zucchini, and Bell Peppers	Harissa Potato Salad	Ricotta & Yogurt Parfait	Baked chicken and Ricotta Meatballs
Day 15	Avocado and Egg Breakfast Pizza	Greek Lemon Chicken Soup	Mediterranean Picnic Snacks	Chickpea Vegetable Coconut Curry
Day 16	Mediterranean Breakfast Sandwich	Mediterranean Bento Lunch	Crock Pot Chunky Monkey Paleo Trail Mix Recipe	Broccoli Rabe and Burrata with Lemon
Day 17	Breakfast Hash with Brussels sprouts and Sweet Potatoes	Greek Meatball Mezze Bowls	Savory Feta Spinach and Sweet Red Pepper Muffins	Tomato Poached Cod with Special Herbs
Day 18	Mediterranean Keto Low Carb Egg Muffins with Ham	Mediterranean Chicken with Orzo Salad	Smoked Salmon, Avocado and Cucumber Bites	Chickpea Shawarma Salad
Day 19	Spinach and Artichoke Frittata	Mediterranean Chickpea Quinoa Bowl	15 Minute Mediterranean Chickpea Salad	Mediterranean Portobello Mushroom Pizzas with Arugula Salad
Day 20	Hearty Breakfast Fruit Salad	Harissa Chickpea Stew With Eggplant and Millet	Lemon Herb Mediterranean Pasta Salad	Slow-Cooker Mediterranean Quinoa with Arugula
Day 21	Shakshuka	Five-Minute Heirloom Tomato Toast	Hummus	Walnut-Rosemary Crusted Salmon

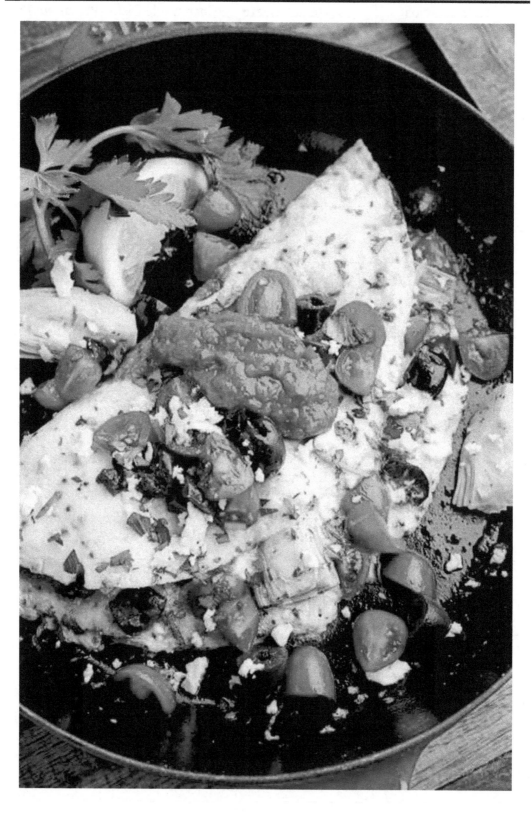

Spinach and Artichoke Frittata

Serving size: 4
Servings per recipe: 2
Calories: 316
Preparation time: 5 minutes
Cooking time: 22 – 25 minutes

Ingredients:

- large eggs 10
- full-fat sour cream ½
- Dijon mustard 1 tbs
- kosher salt 1 tsp
- freshly ground black pepper 1/4 teaspoon
- grated Parmesan cheese (about 3 ounces), divided 1
- cup olive oil 2 tablespoons
- marinated artichoke hearts, drained, patted dry, and quartered About 14 ounces
- baby spinach 5 ounces
- 2 cloves garlic, minced

Nutrition Information: based on 6 servings
Carb: 6.4 g
Protein: 17.9 g
Fats: 25.9 g

Instructions:

- Place a rack in centre of the oven set temperature at 400˚c.
- In a large bowl put sour cream, mustard, pepper salt and half cup of Parmesan cheese, stir with a whisk well until well combined; keep at a side.
- Take a skillet of about 10" skillet (non-stick or cast iron) heat oil over mediuk flame. Put artichoke in a layer, cook stir in between, till light brown, not more than 8 minutes. Now spinach and garlic is to be added, toss it is wilted till liquid evaporates.
- After spreading the mixture evenly in a layer, pour the mixture of egg over vegetables. Sprinkle 1/2 cup of Parmesan. For setting the eggs well over veggies tilt it. Cook for 2-3 minutes or till the time the eggs settle.
- Bake for 13-15 minutes. Cut in the centre of frittata to check even cooking. Leave it for five minutes to cool, slice into wedges shape.

Hearty Breakfast Fruit Salad

Serving size: 1
Servings per recipe: 5
Calories: 282
Preparation time: 10 minutes
Cooking time: 1 hour 20 minutes

Ingredients:

- pearl or hulled barley or any sturdy whole grain 1 cup
- water 3 cups
- olive oil, divided 3 tablespoons
- kosher salt 1/2 teaspoon
- 1/2 large pineapple, peeled and cut into 1 1/2- to 2-inch chunks (2 to 2 1/2 cups)
- medium tangerines or mandarin 6 , or large oranges 5(about 1 1/2 pounds total)
- pomegranate seeds 1 1/4 cups
- small bunch fresh mint 1

For the dressing:

- honey or another sweetener 1/3 cup
- Juice and finely grated zest of 1 lemon (about 1/4 cup juice)
- Juice and finely grated zest of 2 limes (about 1/4 cup juice)
- kosher salt 1/2 teaspoon
- olive oil 1/4 cup
- toased hazelnut or nut oil 1/4 cup

Nutrition Information

Carbs: 34.8 g

Proteins: 3.7 g

Fats: 16.6 g

Instructions

- With a parchment paper line rimmed baking sheets. In a strainer wash barley under cold water till the water below is clear for around one minute. Shake the strainer gently to drain off the excess water. On one of the prepared baking sheets place barley and using spatula spread out the grains into a single layer. Leave it be completely dry for 3-4 minutes.
- In a microwave or stove top warm the water, keep it aside.
- In a medium saucepan heat 2 tablespoon oil on high heat till simmering. Add barely carefully and toast, keep stirring constantly, till they darken a bit. It generally takes 1 minute to 90 seconds.

- Add salt and warm water and bring it to boil. Turn the heat to simmer to the lowest, cover the pan and keep cooking until soft and most of the water has been absorbed, for around 40-50 minutes. Take the pot off the heat and leave it covered for 10 minutes, this way the barley would steam and finish absorbing water. By that time prepare mint, fruit and dressing.
- Into one of the large containers place the pineapple chunks. Peel and cut mandarins, tangerines, or oranges into segments, remove as much of the bitter white pith as possible. Place these fruits in another container, cover and refrigerate. Keep pomegranate seeds in a covered box separately and refrigerate.
- Mince or slice the mint leaves thinly. Keep it in a covered container and refrigerator.
- In a medium bowl whisk juice, honey, zest and salt together. Mizzle in olive oil, nut oil, while whisking constantly until incorporated. You can cover and refrigerate or refrigerate in a jar.
- Shift the cooked barley onto the second prepared baking sheet and spread in a layer evenly. Leave to cool completely. For around 10-20 minutes. Mizzle barley with leftover 1 tablespoon of oil and mix to coat.
- Shift barley to a large container. Cover the container and keep in a refrigerator.

At the time of serving, scoop 2/3 cup of barley into each bowl. In each bowl add six pieces of pineapple, 10-12 orange segments, and with it ¼ cup pomegranate seeds into each bowl. Now add 1-2 tablespoons of the mint and 2-3 tablespoons of dressing to each bowl. Stir in order to mix and coat it with the dressing.

Shakshuka

Serving size: 4
Servings per recipe: 6
Calories: 146
Preparation time: 10
Cooking time: 25 to 30 minutes

Ingredients:

- *whole peeled tomatoes 1 (28-ounce) can*
- *olive oil 2 tablespoons*
- *finely chopped small yellow onion 1*
- *tomato paste 2 tablespoons*
- *Harissa 1 tablespoon*
- *garlic, minced 3 cloves*
- *ground cumin 1 teaspoon*
- *kosher salt 1/2 teaspoon*
- *large eggs 6*
- *loosely packed chopped fresh cilantro leaves and tender stems 1/4 cup feta cheese, crumbled (about 1/2 cup, optional 2 ounces*

Nutrition Information based on 10 servings
Carb: 7.8 g
Protein: 7.9 g
Fats: 9.7 g

Instructions

- ✓ In a large bowl pour tomatoes as well as their juice. Crush with hands carefully, pieces should be bite-sized.
- ✓ In a skillet heat oil for 10-12 minutes on medium flame. Now add onion sauté for 5 minutes or till soft. Put harissa, garlic, cumin, tomato paste and salt. Sauté until aromatic.
- ✓ After adding tomatoes simmer till sauce gets slightly thickens. (10 minutes)
- ✓ Now remove skillet from stove. Make small six holes in sauce and crack an egg into each.
- ✓ Spoon a little sauce over each egg. If you expose the yolks, white of egg cooks faster.
- ✓ For even cooking of eggs keep rotating the pan or till the time white sets. It generally takes 8 to 12 minutes.
  Remove the pan from flame. Sprinkle feta and cilantro. Your dish is ready to be served with bread or fita.

Caprese Avocado Toast

Serving size: 2
Servings per recipe: 2
Calories: 649
Preparation time: 4 minutes
Cooking time: 7-8 minutes

Ingredients:

- slices hearty sandwich bread, such as peasant bread, sourdough, whole-wheat or multi-grain- 2
- medium avocado, halved and pit removed- 1
- grape tomatoes, halved- 8
- fresh *ciliegine* or bite-sized mozzarella balls 2 ounces (about 12)
- large fresh basil leaves, torn 4

  balsamic glaze 2 tablespoons

Nutrition Information
Carb: 86.4 g
Protein: 23.9 g
Fats: 24.6 g

Instructions

- ✓ First toaste the bread. Meanwhile mash avocado in a small-sized bowl.
- ✓ Over the toast mashed spread avocado. Use tomatoes, mozzarella balls and basil leaves for topping each slice. Thereafter sprinkle balsamic glaze. Serve at once.

Spinach Feta Breakfast Wraps

Serving size: 4
Servings per recipe: 4
Calories: 543
Preparation time: 10 minutes
Cooking time: 12 minutes

Ingredients:

- large eggs 10
- baby spinach 1/2 pound
- whole-wheat tortillas 4
- cherry or grape tomatoes, halved 1/2 pint
- feta cheese, crumbled 4 ounces
- Butter or olive oil   1 teaspoon
- Salt   ¼ tsp.
- Pepper   ¼ tsp.

Nutrition Information 4 servings
Carbs: 46.5 g
Protein: 28.1 g
Fats: 27 g

Instructions:

- ✓ Stir the eggs well to combine the white and yolks. Coat skillet's bottom with teaspoon of olive oil and place on medium flame. At the melting of butter or heating of oil drain the eggs in skillet, stir in between till the eggs are cooked. Add a pinch of salt with black pepper. Slide the material to a platter, cool at room temperature.

- ✓ Rinse the skillet, now put it on medium flame, and add another teaspoon of oil or butter. Add spinach. Keep stirring until the spinach is limp. Spread wilted spinach on a plate, cool it at room temperature.

- ✓ On a surface arrange a tortilla. Add spinach, tomatoes, feta and quarter of the eggs in mid of tortilla, wrap tightly. Repeat the same procedure with the rest of the tortillas. In a gallon zip-top bag place the wraps and freeze till ready to eat.

- ✓ If you want to freeze longer than a week. In an aluminium foil wrap burritos, it will prevent the freezer from burning. Reheat in microwave on high for 2 minutes.

Easy Homemade Muesli

Serving size: 1
Servings per recipe: 8
Calories: 275
Preparation time: 15 minutes
Cooking time: 15 minutes

Ingredients:

- rolled oats- 3 1/2 cups
- wheat bran- 1/2 cup
- kosher salt- 1/2 teaspoon
- ground cinnamon- 1/2 teaspoon
- sliced almonds- 1/2 cup
- raw pecans, coarsely chopped- 1/4 cup
- raw pepitas (shelled pumpkin seeds)- 1/4 cup
- unsweetened coconut flakes-1/2 cup
- dried apricots, coarsely chopped-1/4 cup
- dried cherries-1/4 cup

Nutrition Information: Carbs: 36 g; Protein: 8.5 g; Fats: 13.4 g

Instructions

- ✓   To divide the oven into thirds, arrange two racks and heat to 350 °F. Put wheat bran, salt, cinnamon and oats on a rimmed baking sheet. Spread an even layer. On the second rimmed baking sheet put pecans, pepitas, and almonds, to combine toss, spread evenly in a layer. Both baking sheets should be transferred to oven, keeping oats on top part of the rack and at bottom nuts.

- ✓   Set aside the baking sheet having nuts in order to cool. Spatter coconut powder over oats. Bake the upper rack till coconut is golden brown, preferably 5 minutes. Remove from, cool for 10 minutes.
  Shift the material of both the baking sheets into a large bowl.
  Put cherries and apricots, to combine well; toss.
  You can store muesli in airtight container at room temperature for a month.

- ✓   You can have it with cereals, yogurt, and oatmeal or with drops of honey.

Kale and Goat Cheese Frittata Cups

Serving size: 1 cup
Servings per recipe: 8 cups
Calories: 179
Preparation time: 5 minutes
Cooking time: 35-40 minutes

Ingredients:

- chopped lacinato kale 2 cups
- garlic clove, thinly sliced 1
- olive oil 3 tablespoons
- red pepper flakes 1/4 teaspoon
- large eggs 8
- Salt 1/4 teaspoon
- ground black pepper Dash
- dried thyme 1/2 teaspoon
- goat cheese, crumbled 1/4 cup

Nutrition Information

Carbs: 1.2 g

Protein: 10.0 g

Fats: 14.7 g

Instructions

- ✓ Oven is to be preheated to 350°F. Remove the leaves from kale ribs for getting to cups of kale. Now wash and leave the leaves to dry. Next cut these leaves into half inch wide strips.
- ✓ Cook garlic in a non-tick skillet, preferably of 10 inch, in one tablespoon of oil. Keep the flame at medium to high level for 30 seconds. Now add kale and red pepper flakes, keep cook until soft. Generally it takes around 2 minutes.
- ✓ Beat eggs along with salt and pepper in a medium sized bowl. Now thyme and kale are to be added to the blended mixture.
- ✓ Grease a 12 cup muffin tin with 2 tablespoon olive oil. The tops are to be spattered with goat cheese. Bake for 25-30 minutes or these are set in the centre.
- ✓ It tastes best if eaten warm. You can refrigerate the leftovers. But consume within a week.

Easy, Fluffy Lemon Ricotta Pancakes

Serving size: 4
Servings per recipe: 12
Calories: 344
Preparation time: 10 minutes
Cooking time: 15-18 minutes

Ingredients:

- large eggs 4
- medium lemon 1
- whole-milk ricotta cheese 1 cup
- whole or 2% milk 1/2 cup
- all-purpose flour 1 cup
- granulated sugar 1 tablespoon
- baking powder 1 teaspoon
- kosher salt 1/4 teaspoon
- Unsalted butter, for cooking 1 tablespoon

Nutrition Information

Carbs: 32.3 g

Protein: 17.7 g

Fats: 15.9 g

Instructions

- ✓ Mix white and yolk of the 4 large eggs with an electric hand mixer in a medium sized bowl.
- ✓ Grate zest and a medium sized lemon over the yolks, squeeze lemon juice into the bowl. Now add 1/2 whole or 2 % milk, 1 cup whole-milk ricotta cheese, whisk to combine. Next add 1 cup all-purpose flour, 1 teaspoon baking powder, sugar (granulated) ¼ teaspoon kosher salt, and mix well to combine.
- ✓ On mid-high speed beat egg whites until stiff peaks form. 1/3 of beaten egg whites stirred into yolk batter using rubber spatula. Gently fold the left egg whites to combine well.
- ✓ On medium flame heat a non-stick skillet. Coat with 1 teaspoon unsalted butter. Put batter into pan ¼ of cup, at a time 3. You can use spatula to spread a round of 4" each. Keep cooking till the surface bubbles appear, edges look dry and bottom turns golden brown, flip and cook till it is golden brown.
- ✓ Pancakes can now be transferred to a warm plate or oven.

Smashed Egg Toasts with Herby Lemon Yogurt

Serving size: 4
Servings per recipe: 4
Calories: 437
Preparation time: 5 minutes
Cooking time: 15 minutes

Ingredients:

- large eggs 8
- garlic 1 clove
- medium lemon 1
- finely chopped fresh basil leaves, plus more for garnish 2 tablespoons
- finely chopped fresh dill, plus more for garnish 2 tablespoons finely
- chopped fresh chives, plus more for garnish 2 tablespoons plain
- Greek yogurt 2 cups
  extra-virgin olive oil, plus more for drizzling 2
- tablespoons kosher salt, plus more for sprinkling 3/4
- teaspoon
- freshly ground black pepper, plus more for sprinkling 1/2
- teaspoon country or sourdough bread (about 1-inch thick) 4 large
- slices unsalted butter, divided 4 tablespoons

Nutrition Information: **Carbs:** 7.4 g; **Protein:** 23.5 g; **Fats:** 35.5 g

Instructions

- ✓ Fill quarter of a large pan with water, boil on high flame, fill another large bowl with ice and cold water. Lower heat to simmer. Lower 8 eggs gently, one at a time. Boil for 6.30 minutes. Now transfer eggs to ice bath, after 2 minutes, peel eggs under running water.
- ✓ Grate the zest 1 medium sized lemon finely, squeeze and extract juice, mince garlic clove. Chop basil leaf to have 2 tablespoon leaves and same amount of fresh dill and fresh chives. Add 2 cups yogurt (Greek) and 2 tablespoon extra-virgin olive oil, ¾ teaspoon kosher salt and ½ teaspoon black pepper. Whisk to combine.
- ✓ Cut 4 slices (1") of a crusty bread. Melt 2 tablespoon unsalted butter in skillet of large size on medium flame. Add 2 slices, cook till crisp and golden brown. Shift to a large platter.
- ✓ On bread slices spread yogurt mixture, top with 2 eggs. With back of a spoon, gently smash eggs. Spatter black pepper, kosher salt and herbs, you can sprinkle a little more olive oil.

Mediterranean Breakfast Pitas

Serving size: 1 filled pita
Servings per recipe: 4
Calories: 206
Preparation time: 5 minutes
Cooking time: 15 -20 minutes

Ingredients:

- large eggs, at room temperature- 4
- Salt to taste
- whole-wheat pita breads with pockets, cut in half 1/2 cup
- hummus 1 (4 ounces)
- medium cucumber, thinly sliced into rounds 2
- large dice medium tomatoes,
- fresh parsley leaves, coarsely chopped Handful
- Freshly ground black pepper
- Hot sauce (optional)

Nutrition Information
Carbs: 22.9 g
Proteins: 12 g
Fats: 8.3 g

Instructions

- ✓ Pour water in medium sized pan to the full. Bring water to boil. Place room temperature eggs in this water and cook for around 7 minutes. Next drain the hot water and place the eggs under running tap of cold water. Now peel these eggs and make slices of ¼ inch thickness. Sprinkle salt.
- ✓ Now spread 2 tablespoons of hummus inside each pita. Now put diced tomatoes and cucumber slices into every pita. Salt and pepper are to be sprinkled now. In each pita tuck a sliced egg and sprinkle with hot sauce and parsley.

Crispy White Beans with Greens and Poached Egg

Serving size: 4
Servings per recipe: 2
Calories: 301
Preparation time: 5 minutes
Cooking time: 15 minutes

Ingredients:

- olive oil, divided 3 tablespoons
- can cannellini beans, drained and rinsed 1 (15-ounce)
- kosher salt, divided 1 teaspoon
- za'atar, divided 2 teaspoons
- medium bunch Swiss chard (about 10 ounces), stems removed and leaves thinly sliced- 1
- garlic, minced 2 cloves
- red pepper flakes, plus more for serving 1/4
- teaspoon freshly squeezed lemon juice 1 tablespoon
- large eggs, poached 4

Nutrition Information
Carbs: 26.5 g
Proteins: 15.5 g
Fats: 15.5 g

Instructions

- ✓ In a large frying pan heat 2 tablespoon oil over medium heat. Keep until shimmering. Spread the beans into an even layer, cook until light brown at bottom. it generally takes 2-4 minutes. Add 1 teaspoon za'tar and ½ teaspoon salt. Stir to combine. Beans are to be spread again and cooked, keep stirring till beans turn golden brown and bubbled on all sides.
- ✓ Put rest of 1 tablespoon oil on the pan. Add chard, rest of half teaspoon salt and 1 teaspoon za'tar, red pepper flakes and garlic. Stir in between and keep cooking until the chard gets soft. Take the pan off the flame, put lemon juice, to combine well toss.
- ✓ In 4 bowls divide beans and greens, top each with a poached egg and a bit more of red pepper flakes.

Breakfast Grain Salad with Blueberries, Hazelnuts & Lemon

Serving size: 2
Servings per recipe: 8
Calories: 353
Preparation time: 5 minutes
Cooking time: 25 minutes

Ingredients:

- steel-cut oats 1 cup
- dry golden quinoa 1 cup
- dry millet 1/2 cup
- olive oil, divided 3 tablespoons
- piece fresh ginger, peeled and cut into coins- 1 (1-inch)
- large lemons, zest and juice 2
- maple syrup 1/2 cup
- Greek yogurt (or soy yogurt, if you want to make this vegan) 1 cup
- Nutmeg 1/4 teaspoon
- hazelnuts, roughly chopped and toasted 2 cups
- blueberries or mixed berries   2 cups

Nutrition Information

Carbs: 38 g

Proteins: 9.3 g

Fats: 20.1 g

Instructions

- √ In a fine mesh strainer mix millet, oats and quinoa. For a minute rinse under running water. Keep aside.
- √ Over medium flame in a 3 quart saucepan heat one tablespoon olive oil. Put rinsed millet, oats and quinoa. Cook for 2-3 minutes. Add 4 ½ cups of water and stir ¾ salt, zest of a lemon and ginger coins.
- √ Bring the water to boil, after covering turn the heat down and simmer for about 20 minutes. Turn the burner off and leave for 5 minutes, remove the lid and touch lightly with a fork. Take the ginger off. On a large baking sheet spread grains allow it cool for minimum half an hour.
- √ With a spoon put the cooled grain into a large bowl. The zest of second lemon is stirred in.
- √ Whisk the remaining olive oil (2 tablespoons) in a mid-sized bowl with juice of 2 lemons, wait till emulsified. Mix yogurt, maple syrup and nutmeg. Flow this into grains and stir unit coated well. Add in blueberries and hazelnuts. Try taste and flavour with salt, if required. For better flavour refrigerate overnight.

Eggs with Summer Tomatoes, Zucchini, and Bell Peppers

Serving size: 1
Servings per recipe: 2
Calories: 226
Preparation time: 5 minutes
Cooking time: 30-35 minutes

Ingredients:

- olive oil 1 tablespoon
- small yellow onion, halved and thinly sliced 1
- garlic, minced 1 clove
- medium summer squash or zucchini (approximately 4 cups) 2
- medium tomatoes, chopped (approximately 3 cups) 2
- fresh thyme (optional) 1/2 teaspoon
- ground Spanish piquillo pepper or Spanish paprika 1 teaspoon
- medium red bell pepper 1
- Salt and pepper 1 tablespoon each
- large eggs 2

Nutrition Information based on 2 serving

Carbs: 20.6 g

Proteins: 11.1 g

Fats: 12.5 g

Instructions

- ✓ In a large heavy skillet heat olive oil at medium heat. Add sliced onions, keep stirring to the point translucence. Next put garlic and cook for a minute. Next add squash and cook for 10 minutes or till soft. Then add, thyme (optional) and piquillo and allow to simmer to the point of even cooking and it turns stewy, for around 20 minutes.

- ✓ Keep cooking ratatouille, meanwhile on the stovetop roast the pepper. Once cool, take off the core and seed, cut into 1'' pieces. Now put the skillet off the flame, add roasted peppers and put pepper and salt as per your taste. It is best to serve the dish warm.

  You fry or boil eggs as per your choice. Divide veggie in two plates and add topping of eggs. You can serve it with buttered toast.

Avocado and Egg Breakfast Pizza

Serving size: 1
Servings per recipe: 4
Calories: 337
Preparation time: 10 minutes
Cooking time: 15 minutes

Ingredients:

- large Hass avocado 1
- finely chopped cilantro 1 tablespoon
- lime juice 1 ½ teaspoons
- salt 1/8 teaspoon
- pizza dough, homemade 1/2 pound
- Large eggs 4
- vegetable oil 1 tablespoon
- Hot sauce, for serving (optional)

Nutrition Information
Carbs: 33.2 g
Proteins: 12.3 g
Fats: 17.6 g

Instructions

- √ Half lengthwise cut avocado, after removing pit, with a spoon scoop the flesh and put into a bowl. Now add lemon juice, cilantro and salt. With a few pieces of avocado, mash using a fork until smooth. Taste and adjust the flavour. If avocado is bigger more salt and lime juice may be required.
- √ Divide dough in 4 pieces of equal size. Now roll each piece into a slim 6" circle. Try again if dough does not stay at a point.
- √ Over a medium flame heat a well-seasoned cast iron skillet. Now place in the centre of the skillet one dough circle. For 1-2 minutes cook or till the underside is brown and the upper side is bubbly. Repeat procedure by flipping the dough circle. Press with spatula if puffing is seen in dough top. It may seem burnt in spots but it's ok. Transfer to platter and repeat with the left dough circles.
- √ On each cooked piece of dough spread the avocado mixture.
- √ Over the medium flame heat oil in the skillet. Now fry eggs to desired level and place it on top of pizza. Serve at once with hot sauce or without it.

Mediterranean Breakfast Sandwich

Serving size: 1
Servings per recipe: 4
Calories: 242
Preparation time: 15 minutes
Cooking time: 5 minutes

Ingredients:

- Multigrain sandwich thins 4
- Olive oil 4 teaspoons
- Snipped fresh rosemary 1 tablespoon or dried rosemary ½ teaspoon
- Eggs 4
- Fresh baby spinach leaves 2 cups
- Medium tomato cut into 8 slices- 1
- Reduced-fat feta cheese 4 tablespoons
- Kosher salt 1/8 teaspoon
- Freshly ground black pepper

Nutrition Information

Carbs: 25 g

Proteins: 13 g

Fats: 11.7 g

Instructions

- ✓ Heat the oven beforehand to 375 degrees F. Now split sandwich thin, next brush cut sides using 2 teaspoons of the olive oil. keep the toast on baking sheet and put in oven for about 5 minutes or till the edges are light brown and crispy.

- ✓ Over medium-high heat 2 teaspoons olive oil and over medium heat the rosemary. Break eggs, one at a time, into skillet. Cook until white are set but yolks are quite runny or for 1 minute. With spatula break yolks. Change side of eggs cook on other side till done. Take off from heat.

- ✓ Now place the bottom half of the toasted sandwich on the 4 serving plates. Divide spinach among sandwich thins on plates. Do toppings of each with tomato slices, an egg, and 1 tablespoon of feta cheese. Sprinkle with pepper and salt. Now top it with the other sandwich thin halves.

Breakfast Hash with Brussels Sprouts and Sweet Potatoes

Serving Size:1
Servings per recipe: 4
Calories: 206
Preparation Time: 10 minutes
Cooking time: 25

Ingredients:

SWEET POTATO & BRUSSELS

- medium-large sweet potato, chopped into bite-size pieces (skin on) -1
- Brussels sprouts (quartered if large, halved if small) 3 cups
- avocado oil (or other neutral oil // or sub water if avoiding oil) 1 Tbsp.
- each sea salt and black pepper- 1 healthy pinch

THE REST

- avocado oil (or other neutral oil // or sub water if avoiding oil) 2 tsp.
- medium yellow, white, or red onion, finely chopped 1/2
- minced garlic cloves , 3
- finely diced Fuji or Jonagold apple (peeling optional // seeds + stem removed) 3/4 cup
- fresh minced sage (or sub dried) 1 Tbsp.
- dried currants (*optional*) 2 Tbsp.
  spicy chicken or pork sausage (*optional* // buy local and organic meat- 1 cup
- whenever possible // or sub <u>Vegan Sausage</u>) fresh spinach-2 heaping cups
- large eggs (farm fresh or organic, free range / pasture raised whenever possible // see notes for vegan options*) -4

Nutrition Information: Carbs: 19.3 g; Protein: 9.7 g; Fats: 11 g

Instruction

- ✓ With a parchment paper line a baking sheet and preheat oven to 400 degrees F.

- ✓ Put Brussels and sweet potato on baking sheet. Mizzle oil, flavour with pepper and salt and toss for coating. Bake for 22-28 minutes. Toss at mid-point for even cooking.

- ✓ By that time over medium flame heat a large skillet. Once it is hot put oil and onion. Sauté for around a minute. Thereafter add apple, garlic, sage and currants. Sauté for around 3 minutes or to the point of turning golden brown and aromatic—stir in-between.

- ✓ Add sausage and keep sautéing till golden brown and thoroughly cooked—5-8 minutes. Stir constantly and use spoon to break sausage in small pieces.

✓ If sausage is cooked, put spinach, cover skillet and cook for a few minutes until tender. Add in and stir roasted Brussel sprouts and sweet potato. Turn off heat and keep aside until serving.

✓ By that time over a medium flame heat a separate skillet. After it is hot add the number of eggs as per desire.

✓ In the pan crack egg and cook for 3 minutes uncovered, after covering with a lid leave for 1-2 minutes to help the white cook and keep the yolk soft.

✓ Garnish with hot sauce and fresh herbs. Store cooled down leftover kept covered in the fridge for 3-4 days. In freezer in can be kept for a month.

Mediterranean Keto Low Carb Egg Muffins with Ham

Serving size: 2
Servings per recipe: 6
Calories: 109 kcal
Preparation time: 10
Cooking time: 15

Ingredients:

- Slices of thin cut deli ham 9
- Canned roasted red pepper, sliced + additional for garnish 1/2 Cup
- Fresh spinach, minced 1/3 Cup
- Feta cheese, crumbled 1/4 Cup
- Large eggs 5
- Pinch of salt
- Pinch of pepper
- Pesto sauce 1 1/2 Tbsp.
- Fresh basil for garnish

Nutrition information

Carbs: 1.8 g

Protein: 9.3 g

Fats: 6.7 g

Instructions

- ✓ Fore-heat oven to 400 F. profusely spray a muffin tin with cooking spray.
- ✓ With each piece of muffin tin is to be lined with 1.5 pieces of ham, ensure that no place is left for egg mixture to fall out.
- ✓ In the bottom of each muffin tin put a little bit of red pepper.
- ✓ On the top of each red pepper put 1 tablespoon of minced spinach.
- ✓ Do topping of pepper and spinach off with a heaping ½ tablespoon of crumbled feta cheese.
- ✓ Whisk the eggs, salt and pepper. Now divide mixture of eggs equally among 6 muffin tins.
- ✓ Bake till the eggs are puffy and are set for around 15-17 minutes.
- ✓ After removing each cup from the tin of muffin, garnish it with ¼ teaspoon of pesto sauce, additionally, you can ass roasted red pepper slices and fresh basil.

Mediterranean Diet Lunch Recipes

Mediterranean Chickpea Quinoa Bowl

Serving size: 1
Servings per recipe: 4
Calories: 479
Preparation time: 5 minutes
Cooking time: 20 minutes

Ingredients:

- jar roasted red peppers, rinsed- 1 (7 ounce)
- slivered almonds ¼ cup
- extra-virgin olive oil, divided 4 tablespoons
- garlic, minced 1 small clove
- paprika 1 teaspoon
- ground cumin ½ teaspoon
- crushed red pepper ¼ teaspoon (optional)
- cooked quinoa 2 cups
- Kalamata olives, chopped ¼ cup
- finely chopped red onion ¼ cup
- chickpeas, rinsed 15 ounce
- diced cucumber 1 cup
- crumbled feta cheese ¼ cup
- finely chopped fresh parsley 2 tablespoons

Nutrition Information 1 ½ cup
Carbs: 49.5 g

Proteins: 12.7 g

Fats: 24.8 g

Instructions

- ✓ In a mini food processor place garlic, paprika, almonds, 2 tablespoon oil, cumin, crushed red pepper. Keep blending until much smooth.
- ✓ In a medium bowl combine olives, red onion, quinoa and left 2 tablespoon oil.
- ✓ At the time of serving divide quinoa mix into 4 bowls and top each with same amount of cucumber, chickpeas and red pepper sauce. Add parsley and feta.

Tomato Salad with Grilled Halloumi and Herbs

Serving size: 1
Servings per recipe: 4 servings
Calories: 197
Preparation time: 8 minutes
Cooking time: 2 minutes

Ingredients:

- tomatoes, sliced into rounds 1 pound
- lemon ½
- Flaky salt and freshly ground pepper
- Extra-virgin olive oil
- halloumi cheese, sliced into 4 slabs ½ pound
- basil leaves, torn 5
- finely chopped flat-leaf parsley 2 tablespoons

Nutrition Information
Carbs: 8 g
Proteins: 9 g
Fats: 15 g

Instructions

- ✓ On a medium high flame pre-heat a grill or grill pan.
- ✓ On a serving plate arrange tomatoes. Squeeze lemon lightly over them flavour with pepper and flaky salt.
- ✓ Oil the grill grates with oil and add halloumi and cook, turn once or till marks of grill appear and cheese is thoroughly warmed. It generally takes one minute per side. Moisten salad with olive oil. Dot with parsley and basil. Serve at once.

Harissa Chickpea Stew with Eggplant and Millet

Serving size: 1
Servings per recipe: 4
Calories: 600
Preparation time: 35 minutes
Cooking time: 1 hour

Ingredients:

Lemon Herb Chicken

- boneless, skinless chicken breasts 1½ pounds
- extra-virgin olive oil 3 tablespoons
- Zest and juice of 2 lemons
- chopped fresh oregano 1 tablespoon
- chopped fresh dill 1 tablespoon
- chopped fresh parsley 3 tablespoons
- Kosher salt and freshly ground black pepper as per taste

Salad

- Barley 1 cup
- chicken broth 2½ cups
- Zest and juice of 1 lemon
- whole-grain mustard 1 tablespoon
- dried oregano 1 teaspoon
- extra-virgin olive oil ⅓ cup
- Kosher salt and freshly ground black pepper as per taste
- red-leaf lettuce, chopped 2 heads red onion, halved and
- thinly sliced- 1
- cherry tomatoes, sliced 1 pint
- sliced avocados- 2

Nutrition Information

Lemon Herb Chicken

  Carbs: 4 g

  Proteins: 39 g

  Fats: 15 g

Salad

Carbs: 60 g

Protein: 15 g

Fats: 36 g

Instructions:

- √ In a re-sealable plastic bag place the chicken. Whisk olive oil, lemon juice, oregano, parsley, dill and lemon zest in a medium sized bowl. Put this marinade into the bag, seal it and keep in fridge for 30 minutes.
- √ Take a medium saucepan, put chicken broth, barley, and bring it to simmer over medium heat. At simmering, cover it and keep cooking till barley is soft, drain water and reserve.
- √ Whisk mustard, oregano, lemon zest and juice in a medium bowl. Flavour with pepper and salt.
- √ Ready grill for high heat. Take the chicken out from marinade and flavour with pepper and salt.
- √ Keep grilling the chicken until properly charred and thoroughly cooked (10-12 minutes), flip in between as required. Take it off the grill and reserve.
- √ Toss tomatoes, onion and lettuce in a large bowl. Add dressing, it should be toss well for proper coating.

Five-Minute Heirloom Tomato Toast

Serving size: 2
Servings per recipe: 3
Calories: 177
Preparation time: 5 minutes
Cooking time: 10 minutes

Ingredients:

- small heirloom tomato, diced-1
- Persian cucumber, diced-1
- extra-virgin olive oil 1 teaspoon
- dried oregano Pinch
- Kosher salt and freshly ground black pepper as per taste
- low-fat whipped cream cheese 2 teaspoons Trader Joe's
- Whole Grain Crisp bread 2 pieces
- balsamic glaze 1 teaspoon

Nutrition Information

Carbs: 24 g

Proteins: 3 g

Fats: 8 g

Instructions

- ✓ Combine cucumber, olive oil, tomato and oregano in medium sized bowl. Flavour with salt and pepper.
- ✓ On the bread top apply the cream cheese and top it with mixture of tomato and cucumber as well as the balsamic glaze.

Eggplant and Herb Flatbread

Serving size: 2
Servings per recipe: 8
Calories: 297
Preparation time: 5 minute
Cooking time: 1 hour

Ingredients:

- Eggplants 2 lbs
- Garlic cloves- 6
- ground cumin ¼ teaspoon
- paprika ¼ teaspoon
- olive oil 2 tablespoons
- lemon juice 1 tablespoon
- tahini ¼ cup
- Kosher salt to taste

For the Flatbread

-

- pizza dough 1/2 pound (whole wheat)
- scallions sliced on a hard angle 1 bunch
- mint parsley and basil leaves 1 large handful
- lemon juice 1 tablespoon
- Kosher salt and freshly cracked black pepper to taste
- Olive oil
- feta crumbled ½ cup

Nutrition Information: Carbs: 31 g; **Proteins:** 15 g; **Fats:** 12 g

Instructions

- ✓ With a fork prick the eggplant all over. Under the broil roast them until skin is blackened all over and the eggplant is soft. Keep in a bowl and cover with plastic wrap. Keep aside to cool for around 45 minutes.
- ✓ Remove the skin of eggplant and cut the inside, discard skin and keep in a tidy large bowl.
- ✓ Mince garlic finely, add a little salt while mincing to combine. Put the eggplant. Now add olive oil, cumin, paprika and lemon juice stir to combine. Put tahini budge to combine. Check taste and add salt and lemon juice as required.
- ✓ Pre-heat oven to 450 F.
- ✓ Roll the dough into a rectangle about the size of sheet pan on a light floured surface. Shift to an oiled baking sheet, mizzle with olive oil. Bake till it turns golden. After removing from oven apply a thick layer of eggplant mixture.
- ✓ Combine mint, scallions, parsley, basil and scallions in a small bowl. Toss with salt, pepper and lemon juice. Mizzle with olive oil and toss. Now put mixture of herbs over the layer of eggplant. Give a finishing touch with feta. Serve at once.

5-Minute Mediterranean Couscous with Tuna and Pepperoncini

Serving size: 1
Servings per recipe: 4
Calories: 226
Preparation time: 3 minutes
Cooking time: 12 minutes

Ingredients:

Couscous

- chicken broth or water 1 cup
- couscous 1¼ cups
- kosher salt ¾ teaspoon

Accompaniments

- tuna Two 5-ounce oil packed cans
- cherry tomatoes, halved 1 pint
- sliced pepperoncini ½ cup
- chopped fresh parsley ⅓ cup
- capers ¼ cup
- Extra-virgin olive oil, for serving
- Kosher salt and freshly ground black pepper to taste
- quartered lemon 1

Nutrition Information
Carbs: 44 g
Proteins: 8 g
Fats: 1 g

Instructions

- ✓ Bring water or broth to boil in a small pot on medium flame. Take the pot off the pot, stir the couscous and with a lid cover the pot. Leave for 10 minutes.
- ✓ Toss together tomatoes, tuna, pepperoncini, capers and parsley.
- ✓ With a cork fluff the couscous flavour with pepper and salt, and mizzle with olive oil. With a tuna mixture top the couscous. Your dish is ready to be served with lemon wedges.

Pesto Quinoa Bowls With Roasted Veggies and Labneh

Serving size: 1
Servings per recipe: 4
Calories: 862
Preparation time: 10 minutes
Cooking time: 40 minutes

Ingredients:

- large Japanese eggplant, cubed 1
- medium zucchini, cubed-1
- cherry tomatoes, sliced in half 1 pint
- romano (or green) beans Handful
- Extra-virgin olive oil
- Kosher salt and freshly ground black pepper to taste
- quinoa, rinsed 1 cup
- pesto ½ cup (home-made)
- labneh or Greek yogurt 1 cup
- minced garlic clove- 1
- Juice from ½ lemon
  cilantro or parsley (or both!), roughly chopped Handful
-

Nutrition Information: Carbs: 96 g; **Proteins:** 32 g; **Fats:** 42 g

Instructions

✓ Fore-heat oven to 400 ° F. with a parchment paper line large baking sheet. Set up zucchini, eggplant, cherry tomatoes and beans on it. Mizzle olive oil over the vegetables and flavour with pepper and salt. Keep roasting till all the vegetables turn tender or get caramelized. It takes generally 30-40 minutes.

✓ Put quinoa to a medium sized saucepan along with 2 cups of water and a little salt. Bring it to boil, with a lid cover it, reduce flame to simmer and cook for around 15 minutes. After quinoa gets cooked, remove the lid, with a fork fluff it and allow it to cool. After quinoa are cooled a bit, using a pesto toss it.

✓ In a small bowl mix garlic, lemon juice, herbs and labneh.

✓ Set up each bowl by placing quinoa and put up veggies in a row to give rainbow like look. Thereafter add a dollop of labneh on one side.

Greek Yogurt Chicken Salad Stuffed Peppers

Serving size: 1
Servings per recipe: 6
Calories: 116
Preparation time: 30 minutes
Cooking time: 0 minute

Ingredients:

- Greek yogurt ⅔ cup
- Dijon mustard 2 tablespoons
- seasoned rice vinegar 2 tablespoons
- Kosher salt and freshly ground black pepper
- chopped fresh parsley ⅓ cup
- rotisserie chicken, cubed-1
- sliced stalks celery-4
- sliced and divided scallions 1 bunch
- quartered and divided cherry tomatoes, 1 pint
- diced English cucumber, ½
- halved and seeds removed bell peppers- 3

Nutrition Information

Carbs: 16 g

Proteins: 7 g

Fats: 3 g

Instructions

- ✓ Whisk Greek yogurt, mustard and rice vinegar in a medium sized bowl; flavour with pepper and salt. Now stir in parsley.
- ✓ Add celery, chicken and three quarters of tomatoes, scallions and cucumber. Budge well to combine.
- ✓ Among the bell pepper boats divide chicken salad.
- ✓ Dress with remaining tomatoes, scallions and cucumber.

15-Minute Mezze Plate with Toasted Za ' atar Pita Bread

Serving size: 1
Servings per recipe: 4
Calories: 731
Preparation time: 10 minutes
Cooking time: 5 minutes

Ingredients:

- whole-wheat pita rounds 4
- extra-virgin olive oil 4 tablespoons
- za'atar 4 teaspoons
- Greek yogurt 1 cup
- Kosher salt and freshly ground black pepper to taste
- Hummus 1 cup
- marinated artichoke hearts 1 cup
- sliced roasted red peppers 1 cup
- assorted olives 2 cups
- cherry tomatoes 2 cups
- salami 4 ounces

Nutrition Information
Carbs: 62 g
Proteins: 26 g
Fats: 48 g

Instructions

- ✓ Over medium flame heat a large skillet. Each side of pita is to be brushed with olive oil, flavour it with zaátar.
- ✓ Now work in parts, add pita to the skillet and toast till it turns golden brown, for around 2 minutes each side. Cut each pita into quarters.
- ✓ With salt and pepper flavour Greek yogurt.
- ✓ For assembling divide Greek yogurt, artichoke hearts, roasted red, pitas, hummus, tomatoes and salami in four plates.

Greek Lemon Chicken Skewers with Tzatziki Sauce

Serving size: 1
Servings per recipe: 6
Calories: 68
Preparation time: 30 minutes
Cooking time: 1 hour

Ingredients:

TZATZIKI SAUCE

- Greek yogurt 1 cup
- Diced European cucumber- ½
- extra-virgin olive oil 1 tablespoon
- lemon juice 2 tablespoons
- Garlic powder Pinch
- Salt and freshly ground black pepper to taste
- fresh chopped dill ¼ cup

Nutrition Information

Carbs: 3 g

Proteins: 4 g

Fats: 5 g

Instructions

Mix yogurt, olive oil, cucumber, lemon juice and garlic powder in a medium sized bowl. Flavour with pepper and salt and then budge in a dill.

Whisk yogurt with lemon zest, lemon juice, oregano, and cayenne and garlic powder in a small bowl.

Rub the chicken with yogurt-lemon mixture to coat well in a separate bowl.

✓ On each skewer put one piece of chicken, weave the strip back and forth while threading it on to the skewer for securing it.

✓ With olive oil brush both sides of skewers and then flavour with pepper and salt. In batch cook on fore-heated grill or grill pan, char nicely on both side, for 4-5 minutes on each side.

✓ Garnish with tzatziki sauce and parsley. Serve at once.

This Eggplant Pizza is Low-Carb, Gluten-Free and Ready in Under An Hour

Serving Size: 1
Servings per recipe: 6
Calories: 257
Preparation time: 15 minutes
Cooking time: 20 minutes

Ingredients:

- Eggplants-1 large or 2 medium
- olive oil ⅓ cup
- Salt and freshly ground black pepper to taste
- marinara sauce homemade 1¼ cups
- shredded mozzarella cheese 1½ cups
- cherry tomatoes, halved 2 cups
- torn basil leaves ½ cup

Nutrition Information

Carbs: 13 g

Proteins: 8 g

Fats: 20 g

Instructions

- √ Fore-heat oven to 400 °F. With a parchment paper line a baking sheet.
- √ Knife the ends off the eggplant(s) and then cut into ¾ inch-thick slices. Set up these slices on the readied baking sheets. Brush both sides of the slices with olive oil. Flavour with pepper and salt.

3. Roast slices of eggplant until almost tender (10-12 minutes).

4 . Take the trays out from the oven and spread marinara sauce on top of each piece.

Place the pizza in the oven roast till the cheese melts and tomatoes get blistered. (5-7 minutes).

√ Garnish pizza with basil and serve hot.

Wild Alaska Salmon and Smashed Cucumber Grain Bowls

Serving size: 1
Servings per recipe: 4
Calories: 841
Preparation time: 15 minutes
Cooking time: 40 minutes

Ingredients:

- Farro 2 cups
- Juice of 2 lemons
- Dijon mustard 2 tablespoons
- minced garlic clove-1
- extra-virgin olive oil ⅓ cup plus 2 tablespoons
- Kosher salt and freshly ground black pepper to taste
- European cucumber, cut into 1-inch chunks 1
- seasoned rice vinegar ¼ cup
- chopped fresh parsley ¼ cup
- chopped fresh mint ¼ cup

  chopped fresh dill ¼ cup
- Four wild Alaska sockeye salmon fillets 6-ounce

Nutrition Information

Carbs: 69 g

Proteins: 49 g

Fats: 43 g

Instructions

- ✓ Large pot of salted water is brought to boil. Put farro into boiling water. Cook until wilted. (25-30 minutes) Drain.
- ✓ In a medium bowl shift farro. Now mix mustard, garlic, lemon juice and 1/3 cup of olive oil; flavour with pepper and salt.
- ✓ Roughly smash cucumber chunks with large fork in a separate medium sized bowl. After adding rice vinegar toss to combine. Flavour with pepper and salt, add mint, dill and parsley.
- ✓ Heat the remaining 2 tablespoon olive oil in a skillet over medium heat. Flavour salmon with salt and pepper. Next ass fillets to hot oil and keep cooking till the desired level of doneness is attained or 8-10 minutes.
- ✓ Now divide farro into four bowls. Break one salmon fillet in each bowl do topping with herbs and cucumbers.

Harissa Potato Salad

Serving size: 1
Servings per recipe: 4
Calories: 231
Preparation time: 10 minutes
Cooking time: 15 minutes

Ingredients:

- 1 1/2 lbs baby potatoes (leave the skins on)
- 2 tablespoons harissa paste
- 6 ounces low-fat or non-fat Greek yogurt
- 1/4 tsp. salt
- 1/4 tsp. pepper
- Juice of 1 lemon
- 1/4 cup finely diced red onion
- 1/4 cup fresh cilantro or parsley, roughly chopped

Nutrition Information
Carbs: 28 g
Proteins: 3 g
Fats: 12 g

Instructions

- ✓ In a big pot place potatoes cover and add 2" of salted cold water. Bring it to boil on medium flame. Keep cooking potatoes until fork tender. (9-11 minutes). Drain water and keep aside to cool a bit.
- ✓ Whisk harissa, salt pepper, Greek Yogurt and lemon juice in a small bowl.
- ✓ Shift the potatoes to a large bowl. Put dressing gently fold it in until potatoes are well coated. Thereafter, fold carefully in herbs and diced red onion
- ✓ Serve at once warm at room temperature or when chilled.

Greek Lemon Chicken Soup

Serving size: 1
Servings per recipe: 4
Calories: 252.8
Preparation time: 10
Cooking time: 20

Ingredients:

- olive oil, divided 2 tablespoons
- boneless, skinless chicken thighs, cut into 1-inch chunks 1 pound
- Kosher salt and freshly ground black pepper to taste
- minced garlic cloves, 4
- diced onion 1
- peeled and diced carrots, 3
- diced stalks celery, 2
- dried thyme 1/2 teaspoon
- chicken stock 8 cups
- bay leaves 2
- cannellini beans, rinsed and drained 15.5 ounce
- baby spinach 4 cups
- freshly squeezed lemon juice, or more, to taste 2
- tablespoons chopped fresh parsley leaves 2 tablespoons
- chopped fresh dill 2 tablespoons

Nutrition Information: Carbs: 30.7 g; **Proteins**: 24.8 g; **Fats:** 4.4 g

Instructions

- ✓ In a large stockpot or Dutch oven heat 1 tablespoon olive oil over medium flame. Flavour chicken thighs with pepper and salt as per your taste. Put chicken in the stockpot, keep cooking until golden (2-3 minutes) keep aside.
- ✓ Now add 1 tablespoon to stockpot. Add onion, carrots, celery and garlic. Keep cooking until soft, keep stirring in between. Budge thyme until aromatic (1 minute).
- ✓ Whisk in bay leaves and chicken stock. Bring to boil; lower heat stir chicken and cannellini beans, budge occasionally, until slightly thick. (10-15 minutes)
- ✓ Now stir spinach to the point of wilting (for 2 minutes). Budge in parsley, dill and lemon juice; flavour with pepper and salt as per your taste. Serve at once.

Mediterranean Bento Lunch

Serving size: 1 Bento box

Servings per recipe: 1

Calories: 497

Preparation time: 5 minute

Cooking time: 15 minute

Ingredients:

- chickpeas, rinsed ¼ cup
- diced cucumber ¼ cup
- diced tomato ¼ cup
- diced olives 1 tablespoon
- crumbled feta cheese 1 tablespoon
- chopped fresh parsley 1 tablespoon
- hummus 2 tablespoons

- extra-virgin olive oil ½ teaspoon
- red-wine vinegar 1 teaspoon
- grilled turkey breast tenderloin or chicken breast 3 ounces
- grapes 1 cup
- whole-wheat pita bread, quartered- 1

Nutrition information

Carbs: 60. 5 g

Proteins: 36.7 g

Fats: 13.8 g

Instructions

- ✓ In a medium bowl toss tomato, cucumber, chickpeas, feta, parsley, oil, olives and vinegar. Pack this in a medium-sized container.
- ✓ In a medium container place turkey or chicken.
- ✓ Pack hummus in a dip-size container and grapes and pita in small containers.

Greek Meatball Mezze Bowls

Serving size: 2 ½ cups

Serving per recipe: 4

Calories: 392

Preparation time: 10 minutes

Cooking time: 35 minutes

Ingredients:

- frozen chopped spinach, thawed 1 cup
- 93%-lean ground turkey 1 pound
- crumbled feta cheese ½ cup
- garlic powder ½ teaspoon
- dried oregano ½ teaspoon
- salt, divided ⅜ teaspoon
- ground pepper, divided ⅜ teaspoon

- cooked quinoa, cooled 2 cups
- lemon juice 2 tablespoons
- olive oil 1 tablespoon
- chopped parsley ½ cup
- chopped mint 3 tablespoons
- sliced cucumber 2 cups
- cherry tomatoes 1 pint
- tzatziki ¼ cup

Nutrition information

Carbs: 29.3

Protein: 32.4

Fats: 17.2

Instructions

- √ First of all squeeze excess moisture from spinach. In a medium bowl by mixing well combine the spinach with turkey, feta, garlic powder, oregano, 1/8 teaspoon salt and 1/8 pepper. Prepare mixture into 12 meatballs. Over medium flame a large non-stick skillet. Coat it with spray. Take the meatball in batches if required now add to the pan and keep cooking until evenly brown and are not pink anymore in the center, it will take 10-12 minutes. Set the meatballs aside to cool.
- √ Now in a medium bowl combine quinoa, lemon juice, oil, parsley, mint and the remaining ¼ teaspoon salt and pepper each. Each is to be topped with 3 meatballs, ½ cup cucumbers and ½ cup cherry tomatoes.
- √ After this seal the containers and refrigerate for up to 4 days. Now divide tzatziki in 4 small containers and put in the fridge.
- √ Before you serve, shift the meatballs to a microwave-safe container and heat until steaming. Come back to original container and serve with tzatzik

Mediterranean Chicken with Orzo Salad

Serving size: 1/2 Chicken Breast & 1 Cup Orzo Salad

Serving per recipe: 4

Calories: 402

Preparation time: 10 minutes

Cooking time: 40 minutes

Ingredients:

- skinless, boneless chicken breasts (8 ounces each), halved-2
- extra-virgin olive oil, divided 3 tablespoons
- lemon zest 1 teaspoon
- salt, divided ½ teaspoon
- ground pepper, divided ½ teaspoon
- whole-wheat orzo ¾ cup
- thinly sliced baby spinach 2 cups
- chopped cucumber 1 cup
- chopped tomato 1 cup
- chopped red onion ¼ cup
- crumbled feta cheese ¼ cup
- chopped Kalamata olives 2 tablespoons
- lemon juice 2 tablespoons
- garlic clove, grated-1
- chopped fresh oregano 2 teaspoons

Nutrition information: Carbs: 28.3 g; Protein: 32 g; Fats: 27.5 g

Instruction:

- √ Pre-heat oven to 425 degrees F.
- √ First brush chicken with 1 tbsp. oil and sprinkle with lemon zest and ¼ tsp. salt and one tsp. pepper. Put it a baking dish. Keep baking until an instant-read thermometer after insertion shows 165 degrees F, or for 25-30 minutes.
- √ By that time, bring 32 ounces of water to boil in a medium saucepan over high flame. After this add orzo and cook for 8 minutes. Now add spinach and cook for another minutes. Drain and wash with cold water. Drain well and shift to a large bowl. Add tomato, cucumber, onion, olives and feta. Stir to combine.

✓ In a small bowl whisk the remaining 2 tbsp. Oil, garlic, lemon juice, oregano and the remaining ¼ teaspoon salt and pepper each. Now stir everything except 1 tbsp. of the dressing over the chicken. Serve it with salad.

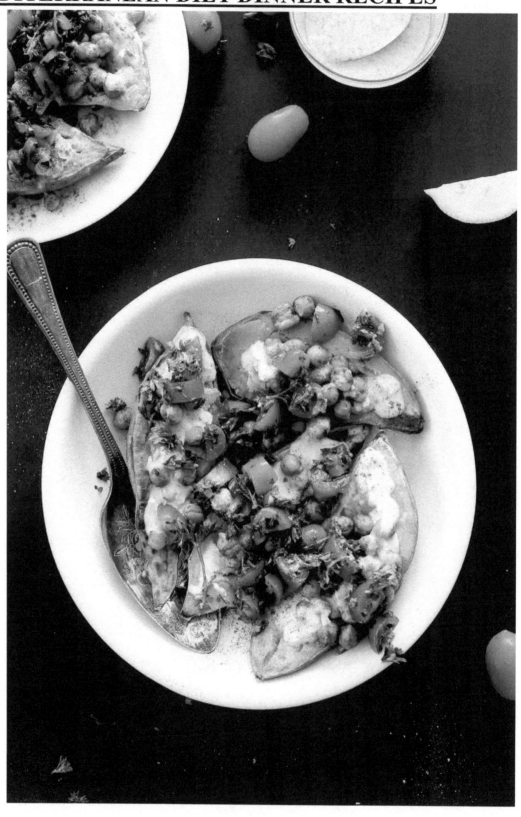

Mediterranean Portobello Mushroom Pizzas with Arugula Salad

Serving size: 1
Servings per recipe: 2
Calories: 264
Preparation time: 10 minutes
Cooking time: 35 minutes

Ingredients:

- large portobello mushroom caps (about 4 oz. each), gills removed 8
- olive oil 2 tablespoons., divided 1 tsp. , divided ground pepper ½
- teaspoon
- pizza or tomato sauce ½ cup
- lightly packed baby spinach, chopped 2 cups sun-
- dried chopped tomatoes ½ cup (about 8) rinsed and
- chopped artichoke hearts, 1 (14 ounce)

Nutrition Information
Carbs: 25 g

Proteins: 14 g

Fats: 13 g

Instructions

- ✓ Fore-heat oven to 400 F°. Use foil to line a large baking sheet and keep it on a wire rack. With 1 tablespoon olive oil brush tops of portobello caps. Now place them undersides-up on the rack. For ten minutes roast. Change side and roast for another 5 minutes.
- ✓ Take out portobellos from the oven and flip them carefully to bring the underside up. Flavour with ¼ teaspoon pepper. Apply 1 tablespoon sauce inside each cap. Divide sun-dried tomatoes, mozzarella and feta among caps. Sprinkle with Italian flavours. Now place portobellos to the oven again and baking to the point when cheese melts and turns brown (10-15 minutes).
- ✓ Whisk the left 1 tablespoon and 1 teaspoon oil and 1/8 teaspoon pepper and lemon juice in a medium sized bowl. Now put arugula and to coat toss.
- ✓ Dress the Portobello pizzas with basil and serve with arugula salad.

Slow-Cooker Mediterranean Quinoa with Arugula

Serving size: 1 ½ cup
Servings per recipe: 6
Calories: 352
Preparation time: 25 minutes
Cooking time: 3-4 hours

Ingredients:

- cups unsalted vegetable stock 2 ¼
- uncooked quinoa, rinsed 1 ½ cups
- sliced red onions (from 1 onion) 1 cup
- minced garlic cloves, 2 (about 2 teaspoons)
- can no-salt-added chickpeas (garbanzo beans), drained and rinsed 1 (15.5 ounce)
- olive oil 2 ½ tablespoons
- kosher salt ¾ teaspoon
- fresh lemon juice (from one lemon) 2 teaspoons
- drained, chopped roasted red bell peppers (from jar) ½ cup
- baby arugula 4 cups (about 4 ounces)
- feta cheese, crumbled 2 ounces (about 1/2 cup)
- kalamata olives, halved lengthwise 12 pitted
- coarsely chopped fresh oregano 2 tablespoons

Nutrition Information
Carbs: 46 g
Proteins: 12 g
Fats: 13 g

Instructions

✓ In a 5-6 quart slow cooker stir stock, quinoa, garlic, chickpeas, onions, 1 ½ teaspoons of olive oil and ½ teaspoon of salt. Close the cooker lid and cook on low flame until the quinoa is soft and stock is absorbed (3-4 hours).

✓ Turn the slow cooker off. With a fork fluff the quinoa mixture. Now mix lemon juice, remaining 2 tablespoon olive oil and ¼ teaspoon salt with a whisker. Now put the red bell peppers and olive oil into slow cooker. Gently toss to combine and fold in the same manner in the arugula. Keep it this way for 10 minutes or until the arugula is gently wilted. Mizzle each serving evenly with feta cheese, olive oil and oregano.

Walnut-Rosemary Crusted Salmon

Serving size: 3 ounces
Servings per recipe: 4
Calories: 222
Preparation time: 10 minutes
Cooking time: 10 minutes

Ingredients:

- Dijon mustard 2 teaspoons
- minced clove garlic 1
- lemon zest ¼ teaspoon
- lemon juice 1 teaspoon
- chopped fresh rosemary 1 teaspoon
- Honey ½ teaspoon
- kosher salt ½ teaspoon
- crushed red pepper ¼ teaspoon
- panko breadcrumbs 3 tablespoons
- finely chopped walnuts 3 tablespoons
- extra-virgin olive oil 1 teaspoon
- skinless salmon fillet, fresh or frozen 1 (1 pound)
- Olive oil cooking spray 1 serving
- Chopped fresh parsley and lemon wedges for garnish

Nutrition Information

Carbs: 4 g

Proteins: 24 g

Fats: 12 g

Instructions

Fore-heat oven to 425 F°. With a parchment paper line a large rimmed baking sheet. In a small bowl combine lemon juice, lemon zest, mustard, rosemary, honey, salt and crushed red pepper. In another small bowl combine panko, walnuts and oil. On the prepared baking sheet place salmon. Over the fish spread mustard mixture and sprinkle with mixture of panko, press to adhere. With cooking spray coat lightly.

✓ Bake until fish flakes set easily with a fork (8-12 minutes).

✓ Sprinkle with parsley and serve with lemon wedges, if desired.

Mediterranean Stuffed Chicken Breasts

Serving size: ½ breast
Servings per recipe: 8
Calories: 179
Preparation time: 35 minutes
Cooking time: 25 minutes

Ingredients:

- crumbled feta cheese ½ cup
- chopped roasted red bell peppers ½ cup
- chopped fresh spinach ½ cup
- Kalamata olives, pitted and quartered ¼ cup
- chopped fresh basil 1 tablespoon
-
- chopped fresh flat-leaf parsley 1 tablespoon
- minced cloves garlic, 2
- boneless, skinless chicken breasts- 4 (8 ounce)
- salt ¼ teaspoon
- ground pepper ½ teaspoon
- extra-virgin olive oil 1 tablespoon
- lemon juice 1 tablespoon

Nutrition Information

Carbs: 1.9 g

Proteins: 24.4 g

Fats: 7.4 g

Instructions

- ✓ Heat oven beforehand to 400 F, in a medium bowl combine feta, spinach, roasted red peppers, olives, basil, parsley and garlic.

- ✓ To form a pocket cut horizontal slit through the thickest portion of each chicken breast. With 1/3 cup of feta mixture stuff each breast pocket; using wooden picks to secure the pockets. With pepper and salt sprinkle the chicken evenly.

- ✓ In a large oven-safe skillet heat oil over medium flame. Set up stuffed breasts upside down, in the pan, cook until golden, about 2 minutes. Flip the chicken carefully. Shift the pan to the oven. Keep baking until as instant-read thermometer is inserted in the thickest portion of the chicken and shows 165 degrees F (20-25 minutes). Drizzle chicken evenly with lemon juice. Keep in mind that wooden picks from the chicken before serving.

Charred Shrimp & Pesto Buddha Bowls

Serving size: 2 ½ cup
Servings per recipe: 4
Calories: 429
Preparation time: 5 minutes
Cooking time: 20 minutes

Ingredients:

- prepared pesto ⅓ cup
- balsamic vinegar 2 tablespoons
- extra-virgin olive oil 1 tablespoon
- salt ½ teaspoon
- ground pepper ¼ teaspoon
- peeled and deveined large shrimp 1 pound (16-20 count), patted dry
- arugula 4 cups
- cooked quinoa 2 cups
- halved cherry tomatoes 1 cup
- diced avocado-1

Nutrition Information
Carbs: 29.3 g
Proteins: 30.9 g
Fats: 22 g

Instructions

In a large bowl whisk vinegar, pesto, oil, pepper and salt. Shift 4 tablespoons of mixture. Keep both bowls aside.

✓ Over medium flame heat a large cast-iron skillet. Put shrimp and cook stirring till the shrimp gets cooked through and is slightly charred (4-5 minutes) transfer to plate.

✓ In a large bowl add quinoa and arugula with vinaigrette and toss to coat. Divide the arugula mixture between 4 bowls. Do topping with tomatoes, avocado and shrimp. Mizzle each bowl with 1 tablespoon of the reserved pesto mixture.

Sheet-Pan Salmon with Sweet Potatoes & Broccoli

Serving size: 2
Servings per recipe: 4
Calories: 504
Preparation time: 15 minutes
Cooking time: 20 minutes

Ingredients:

- 3 tablespoons low-fat mayonnaise
- 1 teaspoon chili powder
- 2 medium sweet potatoes, peeled and cut into 1-inch cubes
- 4 teaspoons olive oil, divided
- ½ teaspoon salt, divided
- ¼ teaspoon ground pepper, divided
- 4 cups broccoli florets (8 oz.; 1 medium crown)
- 1 ¼ pounds salmon fillet, cut into 4 portions
- 2 limes, 1 zested and juiced, 1 cut into wedges for serving ¼
- cup crumbled feta or cotija cheese ½ cup chopped fresh
- cilantro

Nutrition Information: Carbs: 34 g; Proteins: 34 g; Fats: 26 g

Instructions

- ✓ Fore-heat the oven to 425 degrees F. With a foil line a large rimmed baking sheet and coat with cooking spray.
- ✓ Combine chilli powder and mayonnaise in a small bowl. Keep aside.
- ✓ In a medium bowl toss sweet potatoes with 2 teaspoon oil, ¼ teaspoon salt and 1/8 teaspoon pepper. Spread it on the baking sheet prepared. For 15 minutes roast it.
- ✓ In the same bowl toss broccoli with the remaining 2 teaspoon oil, 1/8 teaspoon pepper ¼ salt. Now remove the baking sheet form the oven. Now stir the sweet potatoes and push them to the sides of the pan. Move salmon in the center of the pan and on either side spread broccoli, among sweet potatoes. Spread 2 tablespoons of mayonnaise mixture over the salmon. Bake for around 15 minutes or until the sweet potatoes are tender and salmon flakes conveniently with a fork.
- ✓ By that time, add lime zest and lemon juice to remaining 1 tablespoon low fat mayonnaise; mix it well.
- ✓ Among 4 plates divide salmon and top with cheese and cilantro. Divide the broccoli and the sweet potatoes among the plates mizzle with the lime-mayonnaise sauce. You can serve with wedges of lime and any leftover sauce.

Greek Cauliflower Rice Bowls with Grilled Chicken

Serving size: 4
Servings per recipe: 2
Calories: 411
Preparation time: 5 minutes
Cooking time: 30 minutes

Ingredients:

- extra-virgin olive oil, divided 6 tablespoons plus 1 teaspoon
- cauliflower rice 4 cups
- chopped red onion ⅓ cup
- salt, divided ¾ teaspoon
- chopped fresh dill, divided ½ cup
- boneless, skinless chicken breasts 1 pound
- ground pepper, divided ½ teaspoon
- 3 tablespoons lemon juice
- dried oregano 1 teaspoon
- halved cherry tomatoes 1 cup
- chopped cucumber 1 cup
- 2 tablespoons chopped Kalamata olives
- 2 tablespoons crumbled feta cheese
- 4 wedges Lemon wedges for serving

Nutrition Information: Carbs: 29 g; Proteins: 9.5 g; Fats: 27 g

Instructions

1.   Fore-heat grill to medium

2.   Over medium high flame heat 2 tablespoon oil in a large skillet. Cook for about 5 minutes or until the cauliflower is softened, stir occasionally. Remove from heat and dodge in ¼ cup dill.

3.   Rub 1 teaspoon oil all over chicken. Sprinkle ¼ teaspoon pepper and ¼ teaspoon salt. Flip and grill, check using an instant-read thermometer into the thickest part of the breast. It should show temperature of 165 degrees (15 minutes total) cut in crosswise slices.

4.   In a small bowl whisk remaining 4 tablespoons oil, lemon juice, oregano and the ¼ teaspoon salt and pepper.

5.   Do part cauliflower rice in four bowls. Top with tomatoes, cucumber, chicken, olives and feta. Sprinkle remaining ¼ cup dill. Mizzle vinaigrette. You can serve with lemon wedges.

Prosciutto Pizza with Corn & Arugula

Serving size: ¼ pizza
Servings per recipe: 4
Calories: 436
Preparation time: 10 minutes
Cooking time: 20 minutes
Ingredients:

- pizza dough, preferably whole-wheat 1 pound
- extra-virgin olive oil, divided 2 tablespoons
- minced clove garlic, 1
- part-skim shredded mozzarella cheese 1 cup
- fresh corn kernels 1 cup
- very thinly sliced prosciutto, torn into 1-inch pieces 1 ounce
- arugula 1 ½ cups
- torn fresh basil ½ cup
- ground pepper ¼ teaspoon

Nutrition Information (per serving)
Carbs: 53.1 g
Proteins: 18.3 g
Fats: 19.9 g

Instructions

✓ Fore-heat grill to medium-high flame.

✓ On a lightly floured surface roll dough into a 12" oval. Shift it to a lightly floured baking sheet. In a small bowl combine 1 tablespoon oil and garlic. Bring the garlic oil, cheese, dough, corn and prosciutto to the grill.

✓ Apply oil on the grill rack. Shift the crust to the grill. Keep grilling the dough until it gets puffed and turn slightly brown (1-2 minutes).

✓ Turn the crust over and apply garlic oil on it. top with corn, cheese and prosciutto. Grill, covering it, unit the cheese is melted and the crust is lightly brown at bottom or 2-3 minutes more. Put the pizza back on the baking sheet.

✓ Do topping of the pizza with basil, arugula, basil and pepper. Mizzle with the leftover tablespoon oil.

Vegan Mediterranean Lentil Soup

Serving size: 1 cup
Servings per recipe: 6
Calories: 272
Preparation time: 20 minutes
Cooking time: 40 minutes

Ingredients:

- extra-virgin olive oil 2 tablespoons
- chopped yellow onions 1 ½ cups
- chopped carrots 1 cup
- minced garlic, 3 cloves
- no-salt-added tomato paste 2 tablespoons
- reduced-sodium vegetable broth 4 cups
- Water 1 cup
- no-salt-added cannellini beans, rinsed- 1 (15 ounce)
- mixed dry lentils (brown, green and black) 1 cup
- chopped sun-dried tomatoes in oil, drained ½ cup
- Salt ¾ teaspoon
- ground pepper ½ teaspoon
- chopped fresh dill, plus more for garnish 1 tablespoon
- red-wine vinegar 1 ½ teaspoons

Nutrition Information

Carbs: 42 g

Proteins: 13 g

Fats: 7 g

Instructions

✓ In a large heavy pot heat oil on medium flame. Add carrots and onion; cook stirring in between, until soft (3-4 minutes). Next add garlic and cook stirring constantly, until mixture is coated evenly, about 1 minutes.

Stir in broth, water, cannellini beans, lentils, sun-dried tomatoes, salt and pepper. Bring to a boil over medium-high heat; reduce heat to medium-low. After covering let it summer until lentil turn soft 30-40 minutes.

3. Take off from flame and stir in vinegar and dill. You can add additional dill as per your taste.

BBQ Shrimp with Garlicky Kale & Parmesan-Herb Couscous

Serving size: 3 Oz. Shrimp, 1 Cup Kale & 1/2 Cup Couscous Each
Servings per recipe: 4
Calories: 414
Preparation time: 10 minutes
Cooking time: 20 minutes

Ingredients:

- low-sodium chicken broth 1 cup
- poultry seasoning ¼ teaspoon
- whole-wheat couscous ⅔ cup
- grated Parmesan cheese ⅓ cup
- butter 1 tablespoon
  extra-virgin olive oil, divided 3
- tablespoons
- chopped kale 8 cups

- water ¼ cup
- smashed garlic clove 1 large
- crushed red pepper ¼ teaspoon
- salt ¼ teaspoon
  peeled and deveined raw shrimp 1
- pound (26-30 per pound)
  barbecue sauce ¼ cup

Nutrition Information: Carbs: 36.4 g; **Proteins:** 32.4 g; **Fats:** 16.9 g

Instructions

1.   In a medium size saucepan combine broth and poultry over medium heat. Bring to boil, stir in couscous. Take off from flame and cover the pan leave it for around 5 minutes. With a fork fluff, then stir in Parmesan and butter. Keep it covered so that it stays warm longer.

2.   In a large skillet heat 1 tablespoon oil on medium heat. Add kale and cook for 1-2 minutes or cook until it looks bright green. Now pour water cover the skillet and cook, stirring until kale is soft for about 3 minutes. Bring heat down to medium low. Dig in the center of kale and add 1 tbps. Oil, garlic and crushed red pepper; cook, constantly for 15 seconds, thereafter, stir the garlic oil into kale and flavour with salt. Shift to a bowl and cover to keep it warm.

Now put tablespoon oil and shrimp to pan. Keep cooking stirring in between until the shrimp are curled and pink (2 minutes) take off from the flame and stir in barbecue sauce. Serve the shrimp with couscous and kale.

Green Shakshuka with Spinach, Chard & Feta

Serving size: 1 Egg & 1/2 Cup Greens
Servings per recipe: 6
Calories: 296
Preparation time: 10 minutes
Cooking time: 20 minutes

Ingredients:

- extra-virgin olive oil ⅓ cup
- finely chopped large onion, 1
- chard, stemmed and chopped 12 ounces
- mature spinach, stemmed and chopped 12 ounces
- dry white wine ½ cup
- small jalapeño or serrano pepper, thinly sliced 1
- cloves garlic, very thinly sliced 2 medium
- kosher salt ¼ teaspoon
- ground pepper ¼ teaspoon low-sodium no-
- chicken or chicken broth ½ cup unsalted butter 2
- tablespoons large eggs- 6
-
- crumbled feta or goat cheese ½ cup

Nutrition Information

Carbs: 8.5 g

Proteins: 10.7 g

Fats: 23.4 g

Instructions

2. In a large skillet heat oil over medium flame. Cook for 7-8 minutes adding onion, stirring in between, until soft and translucent but not brown. Put spinach and chard a few handfuls at a time and cook stirring often until soft. Add wine garlic, jalapeno, garlic, pepper and salt; cook stirring in between to the point wine gets absorbed and the garlic turns wilt. Put butter and broth, cook stirring to the point when butter melts and liquid gets absorbed, 1 to 2 minutes.

3. Crack the eggs over the veggies. Cover the skillet and cook over medium-low flame till the whites are set (3-5 minutes). Take off from flame and dredge with cheese, cover and leave for 2 minutes then serve.

One-Skillet Salmon with Fennel & Sun-Dried Tomato Couscous

Serving size: 4 Oz. Salmon & 1 1/4 Cups Couscous
Servings per recipe: 4
Calories: 543
Preparation time: 10 minutes
Cooking time: 30 minutes

Ingredients:

- Lemon 1

- salmon skinned and cut into 4 portions 1 ¼ pounds salt ¼ teaspoon

- ground pepper ¼ teaspoon sun-dried tomato pesto, divided 4 tablespoons extra-virgin olive oil, divided 2 tablespoons

- fennel bulbs, cut into 1/2-inch wedges; fronds reserved 2 medium Israeli

- couscous, preferably whole-wheat 1 cup scallions, sliced- 3

- low-sodium chicken broth 1 ½ cups

- sliced green olives ¼ cup

- tablespoons toasted pine nuts

- cloves garlic, sliced

Nutrition Information: Carbs: 46 g; **Proteins:** 38.3 g; **Fats:** 7.6 g

Instructions

3. Grate lemon zest and preserve it. Knife 8 slices of lemon. Flavour lemon with pepper and salt. Next apply 1 ½ tsps. Of pesto on each piece.

4. In a large skillet heat 1 tbs. oil over medium flame. For 2-3 minutes cook half the fennel till it turns brown at the bottom. Turn the flame down and repeat with one tbs. oil and fennel. Shift to the plate. In the pan add scallions and couscous, cook stirring frequently, till the couscous turns lightly toasted (1-2 minutes). Stir in broth, pine nuts, olives, garlic, the reserved zest and the leftover two tablespoons of pesto.

5. Take the couscous and nestle fennel and salmon into it. Using lemon slices top the salmon. Turn down the flame to medium low, cook keeping the pan covered till the salmon is thoroughly cooked (10-15 minutes). Dress with fennel fronds, if you wish to do so.

Chicken & Spinach Skillet Pasta with Lemon & Parmesan

Serving size: Scant 2 Cups
Servings per recipe: 4
Calories: 335
Preparation time: 10 minutes
Cooking time: 25 minutes

Ingredients:

- gluten-free whole-wheat penne pasta 8 ounces
- extra-virgin olive oil 2 tablespoons
- boneless, skinless chicken breast or thighs, trimmed, if necessary, and cut into bite-size pieces 1 pound
- salt ½ teaspoon
- ground pepper ¼ teaspoon
- garlic, minced 4 cloves
- dry white wine ½ cup
- Juice and zest of 1 lemon
- chopped fresh spinach 10 cups
- grated Parmesan cheese, divided 4 tablespoons

Nutrition Information
Carbs: 24.9 g
Proteins: 28.7 g
Fats: 12.3 g

Instructions

4. Follow cooking directions given on package to cook pasta.
5. In a large high-sided skillet heat oil. By that time, put chicken, add pepper and salt, cook, stirring now and then, just cook through for 5-7 minutes. Now add garlic cook till aromatic for about 1 minute. Stir in lemon juice, wine, lemon juice and zest. Now bring it to simmer.
6. Remove from flame. Stir in spinach and cooked pasta. Cover the skillet and leave it until the spinach is soft. Divide it in four plate and add toppings over each with 1 tablespoon of Parmesan.

Baked chicken and Ricotta Meatballs

Serving size: 5 balls
Servings per recipe: 4
Calories: 454
Preparation time: 15 minutes
Cooking time: 20 minutes

Ingredients:

- broccolini, rough stems trimmed and thick pieces cut lengthwise 14 ounces (400g)
- ends trimmed and thinly sliced lemon, 1
- extra-virgin olive oil, divided 4 tablespoons Kosher salt
- and freshly ground black pepper to taste crushed red
- pepper flakes, or more if desired ½ teaspoon large egg 1
- grated garlic cloves, 2
- ricotta cheese, drained and lightly salted ¾ cup
- parsley leaves and fine stems, roughly chopped ½
- cup panko breadcrumbs ¾ cup
- ground chicken, preferably dark meat 1 pound
- Juice of 1 lemon
- Grated Parmesan, for sprinkling (optional)

Nutrition Information: Carbs: 20 g; **Proteins:** 36 g; **Fats:** 27 g

Instructions

5. Fore-heat the oven at 425°F

6. Toss the broccoli, lemon slices with 3 tablespoons of the olive oil, salt, red pepper flakes and pepper on a baking sheet. Apply evenly on the baking sheet and keep aside while meatballs are made.

7. Beat the egg, thereafter add the garlic, ricotta, 1 tsp. salt, pepper, parsley and rest of the oil, breadcrumbs and meat, and use with your hands in order to combine it gently (if you do too much mushing will make these items dry and tough.) the pieces of meat should be visible through seasoning. Wet your lightly with water and oil and roll the meat into 20 loose round shaped, a little smaller than golf

balls, use a smaller rolling motion between your hands. The water you used will keep them sticking to your hands. Place large pieces of baking parchment on the counter to make it easy for you to clean.

6. On the baking sheet nestle the meatballs between the broccoli and lemon. Keep baking until the meatballs are brown and get cooked through and the broccoli becomes crispy. It generally takes 15-20 minutes. Shake the baking sheet to move the meatballs and turn the tray around midway to make sure that it gets evenly cooked.

7. Take it out of the oven, squeeze the lemon juice on top and place it doing division across plates. Give a finishing touch with grated parmesan, if you are using the one.

Chickpea Vegetable Coconut Curry

Serving size: 1
Servings per recipe: 4
Calories: 665
Preparation time: 10 minutes
Cooking time: 20 minutes

Ingredients:

- extra-virgin olive oil 1- tablespoon
- thinly sliced red onion-1
- thinly sliced red bell pepper 1
- minced fresh ginger, 1 tablespoon
- minced garlic cloves 3
- small head cauliflower, cut into bite-size florets 1
- chili powder 2 teaspoons
- ground coriander 1 teaspoon

- red curry paste 3 tablespoons
- coconut milk 14-ounce
- halved lime 1
- chickpeas 28-ounce
- frozen peas 1½ cups
- Kosher salt and freshly ground black pepper to taste
- Steamed rice, for serving (optional)
- chopped fresh cilantro ¼ cup
- thinly sliced scallions-4

Nutrition Information; **Carbs:** 80 g; **Proteins** 26 g; **Fats:** 31 g

Instructions

Heat oil over medium flame in a large saucepan. Add onion and bell pepper, sauté till almost tender, for about 5 minutes. Next add garlic and ginger, sauté until aromatic for around 1 minute.

Put cauliflower, toss well so as to combine. Stir in coriander, chili powder, coriander and red curry paste, cook till starts becoming caramelised. It generally takes about a minute.

3. Add coconut milk with a stir and bring it to a simmer on medium low flame. Saucepan should be covered while you continue to simmer until the cauliflower is wilted. It will take 8-10 minutes.

4. Take off the lid and squeeze lemon juice into the curry, stir it well to combine. Now add chickpeas, peas, flavour with pepper and salt. Next bring it back to simmer.

5. It is recommended to serve it with rice and dressing should be done of each portion with a tablespoon of cilantro and 1 tablespoon scallion.

Broccoli Rabe and Burrata with Lemon

Serving size: 1

Servings per recipe: 4

Calories: 198

Preparation time: 2 minutes

Cooking time: 8 minutes

Ingredients:

- broccoli rabe, tips of stems trimmed off 1 bunch
- extra-virgin olive oil, plus more for drizzling 1 to 2 tablespoons
- sliced garlic cloves, 2
- red-pepper flakes ¼ teaspoon
- burrata or fresh mozzarella 4 ounces
- fresh lemon juice ½ tablespoon
- crushed, toasted pistachios 2 tablespoons
- Flaky sea salt, for serving

Nutrition
Carbs: 6 g

Proteins: 11 g

Fats: 15 g

Instructions:

- In a large pot bring salted water to boil. For 3 minutes boil the broccoli rabe, thereafter, drain.
- Heat 1-2 tablespoons of olive oil in a large deep skillet over medium heat. It should cover the bottom of the pan nicely. First stir in garlic and cook for 30 seconds, thereafter stir in red-pepper flakes.
- In the pan add the broccoli and sauté, shaking the pan and gently toss it so that cooking gets done, until tender (specially the stems), 3-5 minutes.
- Take off the broccoli rabe from pan and drain off any excess liquid. On a plate arrange broccoli. Tear the burrata and scatter its pieces among the broccoli rabe. Sparge lemon juice, pistachios and salt. Mizzle with olive oil, if you wish to. Your dish is ready to be served.

Tomato Poached Cod with Special Herbs

Serving size: 1 bowl

Servings per recipe: 4

Calories: 261

Preparation time: 5 minutes

Cooking time: 25 minutes

Ingredients:

- extra-virgin olive oil 2 tablespoons
- thinly sliced shallot, 1
- Kosher salt and freshly ground black pepper to taste
- thinly sliced garlic clove, 1
- crushed red pepper flakes, or more, as desired ½ teaspoon
- crushed tomatoes and their liquid 14-ounce
- low-sodium vegetable stock (or water) 1 cup
- cod fillets Four 5-ounce
- parsley or basil leaves and fine stems, roughly chopped or torn, for sprinkling 1 cup
- Toasted crusty bread, for serving

Nutrition; Carbs: 19 g; Proteins: 30 g; Fats: 8 g

Instructions:

1. In a wide shallow skillet heat oil, till it is shimmering. Add salt and shallot, keep stirring until these get soft. Generally it takes 3 minutes. Add pepper and garlic flakes, keep stirring until aromatic, for about 30 seconds more. Pour in stock and tomatoes and turn the flame high and bring the mixture to boil. Turn the flame down to simmer, keep stirring in between, flavour with salt and pepper. Allow it to cook till tomatoes till liquid slightly. It generally takes 8-10 minutes.
2. Flavour the fish with salt and pepper and put the sauce, adjust the heat to maintain a gentle simmer. Cook and spoon the sauce over fillets occasionally, till the fish is covered. Flakes easily when touched, for about 5 minutes. If these don't submerge fully, turn them over halfway. It may take a little longer to cook thick fillet.
3. Between the serving bowls divide the fish and with a spoon put sauce on the top. Give a finishing touch with pepper and parsley and it should be served with bread for dipping.

Chickpea Shawarma Salad

Serving size: 1 dish
Servings per recipe: 2
Calories: 435
Preparation time: 10 minutes
Cooking time: 20 minutes

Ingredients:

CHICKPEAS
- chickpeas 1. 15-ounce (rinsed, drained and dried in a clean towel)
- olive oil 1 Tablespoon
- cumin 1 heaping teaspoon
- smoked paprika 1/2 heaping teaspoon
- turmeric 1/2 heaping teaspoon
- sea salt 1/2 scant teaspoon
- ground cinnamon 1/2 teaspoon
- ground ginger 1/4 teaspoon
- each black pepper, ground coriander + cardamom 1 pinch

SALAD
- spring mix lettuce 5 ounces (organic when possible)
- cherry tomatoes 10 (chopped // organic when possible)
- red onion 1/4 cup (thinly sliced)
- fresh parsley 3/4 cup
- pita chips 20 (slightly crushed // store-bought or homemade* // gluten-free if GF, or sub gluten-free crackers or cooked quinoa)

DRESSING
- hummus 1/2 cup (**DIY** or store-bought)
- garlic 3 cloves (3 cloves yield ~ 1 1/2 Tablespoon // finely minced or grated)
- dried dill 1 teaspoon (or sub 2 teaspoon fresh dill per 1 teaspoon dried)
- medium lemon, juiced 1 (1 lemon yields ~2 Tablespoon or 30 ml)
- Water (to thin)

Nutrition
- ✓ Carbs: 53.3 g
- ✓ Proteins: 19.3 g
- ✓ Fats: 17.3 g

Instructions

1. Heat oven beforehand 400 degrees F. place a rack in the middle of the oven.

2. To a mixing bowl add washed and dried chickpeas. Put olive oil and flavours, toss mixture to combine. Lightly mash half the chickpeas (leaving the other half whole) with a fork to help them cook faster and sprinkle seasoning more easily.

3. Taste a chickpea and adjust flavour as required. Thereafter set a single layer on a bare baking sheet and bake for 20-22 minutes, or until golden brown and crispy. Then set aside.

4. By that time, do preparation for salad ingredients and to a bowl. Reserve pita chips for later. Keep it aside.

5. For preparing the dressing, add hummus, garlic, dill, and lemon juice to a small mixing bowl and using a whisk to combine it. Thereafter add warm water and keep whisking until pourable.

6. When you want to serve add baked chickpeas and pita chips to the salad and half of dressing. Toss in order to combine.

7. Put in the serving dishes and serve with the remaining dressing items.

8. If you want to have best result, store leftovers separately. It stays for 2-3 days, though best when fresh.

Mediterranean Diet Snacks Recipes

Minute Mediterranean Chickpea Salad

Serving size: 1
Servings per recipe: 4
Calories: 196
Preparation time: 15 minutes
Cooking time: 0 minute

Ingredients:

- Chickpeas 1.15 oz (drained, rinsed and loose shells removed)
- cherry tomatoes halved 1 pint
- finely chopped cucumber 1/2
- sliced black olives 1/4 cup
- herbed feta or plain 1/4 cup
- Juice of 1 lemon
- extra virgin olive oil 2 tbsp
- red wine vinegar 1 tbsp
- fresh parsley finely chopped 1/4 cup
- fresh basil finely chopped 3 tbsp
- garlic powder 1/4 tsp
- Pinch of sea salt and black pepper

Nutrition Information

Carbs: 22g

Proteins: 7 g

Fats: 11 g

Instructions

1. Everything is to be combined in a large bowl, toss well to combine. Your dish is ready to be served.

Lemon Herb Mediterranean Pasta Salad

Serving size: 1
Servings per recipe: 10 g
Calories: 108
Preparation time: 10 minutes
Cooking time: 15 minutes

Ingredients: 12 ounces | 350 grams dry pasta (Penne)

FOR LEMON HERB DRESSING:

- olive oil 1/3 cup
- fresh squeezed lemon juice 2 tablespoons
- red wine vinegar 2 tablespoons
- water 2 tablespoons
- finely chopped fresh parsley 2 tablespoons
- minced garlic , 2 teaspoons
- minced dried oregano , 2 teaspoons
- dried basil 1 teaspoon
- salt 1/2 teaspoon
- Cracked pepper , to taste

FOR SALAD:

- Romaine (or cos) lettuce leaves, washed and dried 4 cups
- large cucumber , diced 1
- avocado , peeled, pitted and chopped 1
- large red pepper (or capsicum), deseeded and cut into thin strips 1/2
- grape or cherry tomatoes, halved 9 ounces (250 grams)
- thinly sliced a red onion , 1/2
- pitted kalamata olives , sliced ½ cup
- sun-dried tomatoes packed in oil , drained 1/3 cup
- crumbled feta cheese 5-6 tablespoons

Nutrition Information: Carbs: 3 g; Proteins: 10 g; Fats: 17.1 g

Instructions

1. In a large pot of salted water boil pasta. Drain in a strainer or colander, thereafter wash under cold water in order to take the heat out. Shift the pasta to a large mixing bowl.
2. When pasta is boiling during that time prepare your dressing. In a large jug whisk together all of the dressing/marinade ingredients.
3. In a salad bowl add all the salad ingredients and pasta, and mizzle with a dressing. All the ingredients should be tossed together till everything is coated evenly in dressing. Season with extra pepper and salt, if you feel like doing it.
4. Serve at once.

Hummus

Serving size: 1 small bowl
Servings per recipe: 8
Calories: 173 kcal
Preparation time: 12 minutes
Cooking time: 8 minutes

Ingredients:

- garlic cloves unpeeled-2
- chickpeas 2 cups (342 g)
- lemon juice ¼ cup (60 ml)
- tahini ⅓ cup (67 g)
- kosher salt ½ teaspoon
- extra-virgin olive oil plus more for drizzling ¼ cup (60 ml)
- paprika for garnish

Nutrition Information

Carbs: 12 g

Proteins: 4 g

Fats: 13 g

Instructions

1. Take a small skillet and heat it over medium heat. Toast garlic to the point of it getting brown, shake pan in between. Peel garlic and set it aside.
2. Now drain the chickpeas, reserve ¼ cup of liquid.
3. Wash the chickpeas under cool water. Remove the outer skin using fingertips. If you feel like you can keep the skin but it may affect the smoothness of your hummus repeatedly.
4. Add ¼ cup of reserved chickpea liquid, tahini and lemon juice in a blender or a food processor.
5. Now process it on high speed for a minute, until it becomes frothy.
6. Add garlic cloves, chickpeas, olive oil and salt.
7. On high speed process for a minute. Scrape the sides down.
8. Next process on high speed till it becomes smooth. It will take about two minutes.
9. Check taste of the hummus. Flavour with more salt if you feel the need.
   10.   Serve without delay. Mizzle with olive oil and sprinkle with paprika.

Mini Greek Pita Pizzas

Serving size: 1 ½ round
Servings per recipe: 12
Calories: 69 kcal
Preparation time: 10 minutes
Cooking time: 15 minutes

Ingredients:

- whole wheat mini pitas or slide buns divided in half 6
- olive oil 1 tbsp.
- homemade or store-bought hummus 1/4 cup
- chopped tomato seeded 1/3 cup
- chopped cucumber 1/3 cup
- chopped kalamata olives 3 tbsp.
- finely chopped red onion 3 tbsp.
- crumbled feta cheese 2 tbsp.

Nutrition Information

Carbs: 9 g

Proteins: 2 g

Fats: 3 g

Instructions

1. Fore-heat oven to 350 degrees F.
2. Split 6 mini whole-wheat pitas or mini slider buns in half, so as to have 12 small rounds. Now place these rounds on a baking sheet.
3. Apply some oil over each pita with a brush.
4. Now put in the oven and bake for 15 minutes or till these are crispy and lightly brown.
5. Take it out from the oven and apply a thin layer of hummus over each round, going right up to the edge.
6. On each top place equal amount of tomato, cucumber, red onion, olives and feta. Serve without delay.

Healthy Avocado Cilantro White Bean Dip

Serving size: 2 cups dip with 2 heaping tablespoon serving
Servings per recipe: 6
Calories: 144 kcal
Preparation time: 10
Cooking time: 0

Ingredients:

- Organics cannellini beans (approx. 15 oz)
- large ripe avocado-1
- sour cream 2 tablespoon
- jalapeno slices 2 tablespoons
- garlic cloves-2
- Fresh spinach 1/2 cup (just grab a handful!)
- fresh lime juice 2-3 tablespoon
- fresh cilantro plus extra to taste 2 tablespoon
- olive oil plus extra to garnish 2 tablespoon
- ground cumin ½ teaspoon
- salt 1/4 teaspoon

Nutrition Information
Carbs: 18 g
Proteins: 6 g
Fats: 5 g

Instructions

1. In a large food processor place all dip ingredients. Keep processing until smooth.
2. It can be served at once or can be covered and refrigerated until ready to use.
3. You can garnish with sliced cherry tomatoes, cilantro and red onions.
4. Serve with veggies, *O* Organics blue Corn Tortilla chips with flax seed, *O* organics Pita crackers.

Homemade Granola Bars Recipe (Gluten-Free, Vegan, Dairy-Free)

Serving size: 1
Servings per recipe: 12 bars
Calories: 209
Preparation time: 5 minutes
Cooking time: 1 hour 15 minutes

Ingredients:

- Dried Mulberries, chopped 1/3 cup
- Dried Strawberries, chopped 1/3 cup
- Raw Cashews, chopped 1/2 cup
- Organic Peanut Butter 1/2 cup
- large ripe bananas, mashed 2
- Raw Sunflower Seeds 1/3 cup
- Organic Hemp Protein Powder 2 tablespoon
- Gluten Free Rolled Oats 1 cup
- °Organic Flaxseed Meal 2 tablespoon

Nutrition Information

Carbs: 20.5 g

Proteins: 8.0 g

Fats: 11.6 g

Instructions

1. Heat oven beforehand to 350 F. Use a parchment paper and line an 8X8 square baking pan.
2. Combine the peanut butter and mashed banana in a medium mixing bowl using a manual mixer or an electric whisk.
3. Now add rest of the ingredients in the bowl. Using a spatula mix the ingredients until these are well combined and homogeneous mixture becomes obtainable. Shift the mixture to the ready baking pan. Press it down with a spatula till it is uniform and flat on all sides.
4. Bake it for around 25-30 minutes. Allow the granola to get cool for minimum 40-45 minutes prior to removing it from pam and cutting into bars. Bars should be wrapped in wax paper and stored in the fridge in an airtight container for up to one week.

Charcuterie Bistro Lunch Box

Serving size: 1 box
Servings per recipe: 1
Calories: 452
Preparation time: 5 minutes
Cooking time: 0 minute

Ingredients:

- prosciutto slice 1
- halved mozzarella stick 1
- halved breadsticks 2
- dates 2
- grapes ½ cup
- large radishes, 2
- halved or 4 slices English cucumber (1/4-inch)

Nutrition Information
✓ **Carbs: 64.7 g**
✓ **Proteins: 16.9 g**
✓ **Fats: 17.1 g**

Instructions

1. Knife prosciutto in half-length wise, thereafter wrap a slice around each portion of cheese, dates, breadsticks, grapes and radishes (or cucumber) in a sealable container which has 4-cup division. Refrigerate till ready to eat.

Hummus, Feta & Bell Pepper Cracker

Serving size: I crisp bread with topping
Servings per recipe: 1
Calories: 136
Preparation time: 10 minutes
Cooking time: 0 minutes

Ingredients:

- Hummus 2 tablespoons

- large crisp bread, 1 (Whole Grain Crisp bread)

- crumbled feta cheese 2 tablespoons

- diced bell pepper 2 tablespoons

Nutrition Information
- ✓ **Carbs: 13.1**
- ✓ **Proteins: 6 g**
- ✓ **Fats: 7.1 g**

Instructions

1. On crisp bread spread hummus. Do topping with cheese and bell pepper.

Tomato-Basil Skewers

Serving size: 1 skewer
Servings per recipe: 16
Calories: 46
Preparation time: 10 minutes
Cooking time: 0

Ingredients:

- small fresh mozzarella balls 16

- fresh basil leaves 16

- cherry tomatoes 16

- Extra-virgin olive oil, to drizzle 1 teaspoon

- Coarse salt & freshly ground pepper 1/ to taste

Nutrition Information
- ✓ **Carbs: 1 g**
- ✓ **Proteins: 2.8**
- ✓ **Fats: 3.3**

Instructions

1. On a small skewers mozzarella, basil and tomatoes.
2. Mizzle with oil and sprinkle with pepper and salt.

Marinated Olives & Feta

Serving size: 2 tablespoons
Servings per recipe: 12
Calories: 73
Preparation time: 10 minutes
Cooking time: 1 hour 10 minutes

Ingredients:

- sliced pitted olives, such as Kalamata or mixed Greek 1 cup
- diced feta cheese, preferably reduced-fat ½ cup extra-virgin
- olive oil 2 tablespoons and juice of 1 lemon 1 Zest
- , sliced cloves garlic-2
- chopped fresh rosemary 1 teaspoon
- crushed red pepper 1 pinch
- Freshly ground pepper to taste

Nutrition Information

- ✓ **Carbs:** 2 g
- ✓ **Proteins:** 1.1 g
- ✓ **Fats:** 6.8 g

Instructions

1. In a medium bowl combine feta, olives, oil, lemon juice, zest, garlic, rosemary, crushed red pepper and black pepper.

Garlic Hummus

Serving size: ¼ cup
Servings per recipe: 8
Calories: ¼ cup
Preparation time: 10 minutes
Cooking time: 0 minutes

Ingredients:

- no-salt-added chickpeas (15 ounce)
- tahini ¼ cup
- extra-virgin olive oil ¼ cup
- lemon juice ¼ cup
- garlic clove 1
- ground cumin 1 teaspoon
- chili powder ½ teaspoon
- salt ½ teaspoon

Nutrition Information
Carbs: 9.7 g
Proteins: 3.7 g
Fats: 11.9 g

Instructions

1. Firstly drain chickpeas, reserve ¼ cup of the liquid. Shift the chickpeas and liquid reserved to a food processor. Now add lemon juice, tahini, oil, garlic, cumin, chilli powder and salt. Keep pureeing for 2-3 minutes or till very smooth.

Ricotta & Yogurt Parfait

Serving size: 1 ¼ cup
Servings per recipe: 1
Calories: 272
Preparation time: 2 minutes
Cooking time: 5 minutes

Ingredients:

- non-fat vanilla Greek yogurt ¾ cup

- part-skim ricotta ¼ cup

- lemon zest ½ teaspoon

- raspberries ¼ cup

- slivered almonds 1 tablespoon

- chia seeds 1 teaspoon

Nutrition Information

- ✓ **Carbs: 25.1 g**
- ✓ **Proteins: 21.7 g**
- ✓ **Fats: 9.6 g**

Instructions

1. In a bowl combine ricotta, yogurt and lemon zest. Do the topping with raspberries, almond and chia seeds.

Mediterranean Picnic Snacks

Serving size: 1 ¼ cup
Servings per recipe: 1
Calories: 197
Preparation time: 2 minutes
Cooking time: 3 minutes

Ingredients:

- Crusty whole-wheat bread slice-1, cut into bite size pieces
- Cherry tomatoes 10
- Sliced aged cheese ¼
  Oil cured olives 6

Nutrition Information
Carbs: 22 g
Proteins: 7.1 g
Fats: 9.1 g

Instructions

In a portable container combine bread pieces, cheese olives and tomatoes.

Crock Pot Chunky Monkey Paleo Trail Mix Recipe

Serving size: ¼ cup
Servings per recipe: 5-6 cups
Calories: 250
Preparation time: 5 minutes
Cooking time: 1 hour 30 minute

Ingredients:

- raw walnuts 2 cup (halves or coarsely chopped)
- raw cashews halves 1 cup (whole almonds work too)
- unsweetened coconut flakes 1 cup (be sure to get big FLAKES not shredded)
- coconut sugar 1/3 cup
- butter (cut in slices) 1– 1.5 tablespoon or at room temp 2 to 3 tablespoon coconut oil to make vegan
- vanilla or butter extract 1 tablespoon
- unsweetened banana chips or freeze dried banana slices 6 ounces
- dark chocolate chips or paleo fudge chunks 1/2 cup to 2/3 cup (we used Enjoy life foods brand)

Nutrition Information
Carbs: 18 g
Proteins: 4 g

Instructions

1. In a crockpot place nuts, coconut, sugar, vanilla, butter slices or coconut oil. Mix all these items and keep on high for 45-60 minutes. Don't forget to stir a few times, check in between to make sure coconut that coconut flakes do not burn. Lower the flame after 45 minutes if flakes cook faster or start turning brown.
2. Turn the flame to low and keep cooking for 20-30 minutes.
3. Take it off and place content of crock pot on parchment paper in order to dry out. Ensure that it is cooled for at the minimum 15 minutes prior to adding the chocolate and banana chips.
4. Now add in chocolate chips and banana chips and mix together.
5. Unsweetened banana chips can optionally be added to cook with coconut/nuts, instead of adding afterwards. But it will need stirring frequently. It must be cooked for 45 minutes only.
6. Store in a zip-lock bag or in an airtight container.

Savory Feta Spinach and Sweet Red Pepper Muffins

Serving size: 2
Servings per recipe: 12
Calories: 240 kcal
Preparation time: 10 minutes
Cooking time: 25 minutes

Ingredients:

- all purpose flour you can substitute partly with whole wheat flour 2 ¾
- cups sugar ¼ cup
- baking powder 2 teaspoons
- paprika 1 teaspoon
- salt ¾ teaspoon
- low fat milk ¾ cup
- extra virgin olive oil ½ cup
- eggs- 2
- fresh spinach 1 ¼ cup - thinly sliced
- crumbled feta ¾ cup
- Florina peppers or other red pepper 1/3 cup (drained and patted dry jarred)

Nutrition Information: Carbs: 13 g; Proteins: 4 g; Fats: 2 g

Instructions

1. Heat oven beforehand at 375 F.
2. Mix the dry ingredients: flour, sugar, baking powder, paprika and salt
3. Mix the olive oil, eggs and milk in another bowl.
4. Now add the wet ingredients to the dry ingredients and keep mixing until blended with a wooden spoon. The dough will become thick.
5. Mix gently after adding feta, spinach and peppers, continue till all ingredients are spread thoroughly in the whole mixture.
6. Now divide mixture in muffin pan that you have lined with cupcake/muffin liners. A silicon muffin tray and grease it with a little olive oil. But the oil should be enough for 12 medium muffins.
7. Next bake it for about 25 minutes. Take it off when toothpick comes out clear when inserted in the muffin.
8. Leave them to cool for 10 minutes and then take off from tray, let them cool a couple of hours before you serve it.

Smoked Salmon, Avocado and Cucumber Bites

Serving size: 3 bites
Servings per recipe: 12 bites
Calories: 46kcal
Preparation time: 2 minutes
Cooking time: 8 minutes

Ingredients:

- medium cucumber 1
- large avocado, peeled and pit removed 1
- lime juice 1/2 tablespoon
- smoked salmon 6 oz
- chives, for garnish
- black pepper, for garnish

Nutrition Information
Carbs: 2 g
Proteins: 2 g
Fats: 3 g

Instructions

1.Using a serrated knife slice the cucumber of about ¼ inch thick and lay flat on a service plate.

2. Next put the avocado and lime juice to a bowl and using a fork to mash until creamy.
3. Now assemble the bites and spread a small quantity of avocado on each cucumber, thereafter do topping with a thin slice of smoked salmon.
4. Now dress each bite with finely chopped chives and cracked black pepper. Serve at once.

Conclusion

Today what we desire the most is neither money nor palatial villas but the happiness by living a healthy life. Moreover, we are ready to pay any price for it and equally ready to follow any workout routine. However hard it may be. It is an established fact that there is a direct relationship in our fitness and the food we it. If this food is more plant-based and has good monosaturated fat along with protein. It is a blessing. If it is time tested, it is even better. This is what we find in Mediterranean diet. Going through all these recipes of diet routine—Breakfast, lunch, dinner and snacks, it becomes clear that there is no space for unhealthy fat, preservatives, refined sugar or flour. As all these food items tax different systems of our body. Further, it does not make a hole in your pocket and the ingredients too are easily available.

In the beginning it may be difficult to switch to Mediterranean diet completely. As it is said change is always difficult. But walking a step at a time can always make it possible. You can do it in the beginning by swapping any meal of the day—breakfast, lunch, dinner or even snacks. This diet will make you feel light and healthy—both physically and mentally. There is a science to it. The Mediterranean diet has little saturated fats or any other unhealthy fats. Its monosaturated fat boosts HDL, that is, the healthy cholesterol and keeps our coronary health strong. This is an input that keeps us on track while we follow this diet. As just by doing cardio alone you may not be able to keep your heart healthy by doing cardiovascular exercise alone. Reduced amount of weight would mean, less possibility of type 2 diabetes.

It is noticeable across all the recipes of the diet of people living in Mediterranean basin that it has either plants or fish. It means it has healthy meat and all natural ingredients that has protein, micro nutrients and fibre that makes our internal biological systems run smoothly. The fibre in it helps in cleaning our internal system and the antioxidants mints and vitamin c, B1, B2 and A rich items like quinoa, the chickpea which is rich in Vitamin D, has calcium etc. really ensures its health value. Similarly, there is a reign of fruits like banana, avocado, sweet potatoes; vegetables like tomato, spinach, broccoli, ginger, mushroom and garlic; dry fruits like pistachio, currants; when it comes to fats, there is only healthy fats that comes from olive oil. And the whole wheat and grains keeps you conscious of being full all through and handle those craving better.

The good news is there are lot many options and recipes that resemble items which decorate our platters today—pizza, muffins, salads, snacks, pitas, yogurt, dips etc. Moreover, one can choose easily among vegan, vegetarian and non-vegetarian. It shows following Mediterranean diet is easy and equally easy is to keep it implemented for long time. But we need to give it a start.

Enjoy Your Meal!